50% OFF CNA Test Prep Course!

By Mometrix

Dear Customer,

We consider it an honor and a privilege that you chose our CNA Study Guide. As a way of showing our appreciation and to help us better serve you, we are offering **50% off our online CNA Prep Course.** Many Certified Nursing Assistant courses are needlessly expensive and don't deliver enough value. With our course, you get access to the best CNA prep material, and you only pay half price.

We have structured our online course to perfectly complement your printed study guide. The CNA Test Prep Course contains **in-depth lessons** that cover all the most important topics, over **400 practice questions** to ensure you feel prepared, more than **300 flashcards** for studying on the go, and over **10 instructional videos.**

Online CNA Prep Course

Topics Covered:

- Physical Care Skills
  - o Body Mechanics
  - o Infection Control
  - o Emergencies
  - o Restorative Skills
- Psychosocial Care Skills
  - o Maslow's Hierarchy of Needs
  - o Age-Related Needs and Abuse
  - o Spiritual and Cultural Needs
- Role of the Nurse Aide
  - o Client Rights
  - o Legal Behavior
  - o Ethical Behavior
  - o Communication
- And More!

Course Features:

- CNA Study Guide
  - o Get access to content from the best reviewed study guide available.
- Track Your Progress
  - o Our customized course allows you to check off content you have studied or feel confident with.
- 6 Full-Length Practice Tests
  - o With 400+ practice questions and lesson reviews, you can test yourself again and again to build confidence.
- CNA Flashcards
  - o Our course includes a flashcard mode consisting of over 300 content cards to help you study.

To receive this discount, visit us at <u>mometrix.com/university/cna</u> or simply scan this QR code with your smartphone. At the checkout page, enter the discount code: **CNA50OFF**

If you have any questions or concerns, please contact us at <u>support@mometrix.com</u>.

SCAN HERE

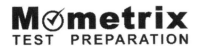
TEST PREPARATION

FREE Study Skills Videos/DVD Offer

Dear Customer,

Thank you for your purchase from Mometrix! We consider it an honor and a privilege that you have purchased our product and we want to ensure your satisfaction.

As part of our ongoing effort to meet the needs of test takers, we have developed a set of Study Skills Videos that we would like to give you for <u>FREE</u>. These videos cover our *best practices* for getting ready for your exam, from how to use our study materials to how to best prepare for the day of the test.

All that we ask is that you email us with feedback that would describe your experience so far with our product. Good, bad, or indifferent, we want to know what you think!

To get your FREE Study Skills Videos, you can use the **QR code** below, or send us an **email** at studyvideos@mometrix.com with *FREE VIDEOS* in the subject line and the following information in the body of the email:

- The name of the product you purchased.
- Your product rating on a scale of 1-5, with 5 being the highest rating.
- Your feedback. It can be long, short, or anything in between. We just want to know your impressions and experience so far with our product. (Good feedback might include how our study material met your needs and ways we might be able to make it even better. You could highlight features that you found helpful or features that you think we should add.)

If you have any questions or concerns, please don't hesitate to contact me directly.

Thanks again!

Sincerely,

Jay Willis
Vice President
jay.willis@mometrix.com
1-800-673-8175

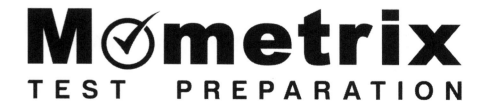

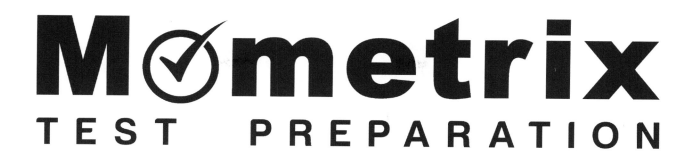

CNA

Study Guide 2023-2024

3 **Full-Length Practice Tests**

Preparation Exam Book Secrets for the Certified Nursing Assistant with Detailed Answer Explanations

5th Edition

Written and edited by Mometrix Test Prep

Printed in the United States of America

This paper meets the requirements of ANSI/NISO Z39.48-1992 (Permanence of Paper).

Mometrix offers volume discount pricing to institutions. For more information or a price quote, please contact our sales department at sales@mometrix.com or 888-248-1219.

Mometrix Media LLC is not affiliated with or endorsed by any official testing organization. All organizational and test names are trademarks of their respective owners.

Paperback
ISBN 13: 978-1-5167-2175-7
ISBN 10: 1-5167-2175-6

DEAR FUTURE EXAM SUCCESS STORY

First of all, **THANK YOU** for purchasing Mometrix study materials!

Second, congratulations! You are one of the few determined test-takers who are committed to doing whatever it takes to excel on your exam. **You have come to the right place.** We developed these study materials with one goal in mind: to deliver you the information you need in a format that's concise and easy to use.

In addition to optimizing your guide for the content of the test, we've outlined our recommended steps for breaking down the preparation process into small, attainable goals so you can make sure you stay on track.

We've also analyzed the entire test-taking process, identifying the most common pitfalls and showing how you can overcome them and be ready for any curveball the test throws you.

Standardized testing is one of the biggest obstacles on your road to success, which only increases the importance of doing well in the high-pressure, high-stakes environment of test day. Your results on this test could have a significant impact on your future, and this guide provides the information and practical advice to help you achieve your full potential on test day.

Your success is our success

We would love to hear from you! If you would like to share the story of your exam success or if you have any questions or comments in regard to our products, please contact us at **800-673-8175** or **support@mometrix.com**.

Thanks again for your business and we wish you continued success!

Sincerely,
The Mometrix Test Preparation Team

Need more help? Check out our flashcards at:
http://MometrixFlashcards.com/CNA

TABLE OF CONTENTS

Introduction

Thank you for purchasing this resource! You have made the choice to prepare yourself for a test that could have a huge impact on your future, and this guide is designed to help you be fully ready for test day. Obviously, it's important to have a solid understanding of the test material, but you also need to be prepared for the unique environment and stressors of the test, so that you can perform to the best of your abilities.

For this purpose, the first section that appears in this guide is the **Secret Keys**. We've devoted countless hours to meticulously researching what works and what doesn't, and we've boiled down our findings to the five most impactful steps you can take to improve your performance on the test. We start at the beginning with study planning and move through the preparation process, all the way to the testing strategies that will help you get the most out of what you know when you're finally sitting in front of the test.

We recommend that you start preparing for your test as far in advance as possible. However, if you've bought this guide as a last-minute study resource and only have a few days before your test, we recommend that you skip over the first two Secret Keys since they address a long-term study plan.

If you struggle with **test anxiety**, we strongly encourage you to check out our recommendations for how you can overcome it. Test anxiety is a formidable foe, but it can be beaten, and we want to make sure you have the tools you need to defeat it.

1

Secret Key #1 – Plan Big, Study Small

There's a lot riding on your performance. If you want to ace this test, you're going to need to keep your skills sharp and the material fresh in your mind. You need a plan that lets you review everything you need to know while still fitting in your schedule. We'll break this strategy down into three categories.

Information Organization

Start with the information you already have: the official test outline. From this, you can make a complete list of all the concepts you need to cover before the test. Organize these concepts into groups that can be studied together, and create a list of any related vocabulary you need to learn so you can brush up on any difficult terms. You'll want to keep this vocabulary list handy once you actually start studying since you may need to add to it along the way.

Time Management

Once you have your set of study concepts, decide how to spread them out over the time you have left before the test. Break your study plan into small, clear goals so you have a manageable task for each day and know exactly what you're doing. Then just focus on one small step at a time. When you manage your time this way, you don't need to spend hours at a time studying. Studying a small block of content for a short period each day helps you retain information better and avoid stressing over how much you have left to do. You can relax knowing that you have a plan to cover everything in time. In order for this strategy to be effective though, you have to start studying early and stick to your schedule. Avoid the exhaustion and futility that comes from last-minute cramming!

Study Environment

The environment you study in has a big impact on your learning. Studying in a coffee shop, while probably more enjoyable, is not likely to be as fruitful as studying in a quiet room. It's important to keep distractions to a minimum. You're only planning to study for a short block of time, so make the most of it. Don't pause to check your phone or get up to find a snack. It's also important to **avoid multitasking**. Research has consistently shown that multitasking will make your studying dramatically less effective. Your study area should also be comfortable and well-lit so you don't have the distraction of straining your eyes or sitting on an uncomfortable chair.

 The time of day you study is also important. You want to be rested and alert. Don't wait until just before bedtime. Study when you'll be most likely to comprehend and remember. Even better, if you know what time of day your test will be, set that time aside for study. That way your brain will be used to working on that subject at that specific time and you'll have a better chance of recalling information.

Finally, it can be helpful to team up with others who are studying for the same test. Your actual studying should be done in as isolated an environment as possible, but the work of organizing the information and setting up the study plan can be divided up. In between study sessions, you can discuss with your teammates the concepts that you're all studying and quiz each other on the details. Just be sure that your teammates are as serious about the test as you are. If you find that your study time is being replaced with social time, you might need to find a new team.

Secret Key #2 – Make Your Studying Count

You're devoting a lot of time and effort to preparing for this test, so you want to be absolutely certain it will pay off. This means doing more than just reading the content and hoping you can remember it on test day. It's important to make every minute of study count. There are two main areas you can focus on to make your studying count.

Retention

It doesn't matter how much time you study if you can't remember the material. You need to make sure you are retaining the concepts. To check your retention of the information you're learning, try recalling it at later times with minimal prompting. Try carrying around flashcards and glance at one or two from time to time or ask a friend who's also studying for the test to quiz you.

To enhance your retention, look for ways to put the information into practice so that you can apply it rather than simply recalling it. If you're using the information in practical ways, it will be much easier to remember. Similarly, it helps to solidify a concept in your mind if you're not only reading it to yourself but also explaining it to someone else. Ask a friend to let you teach them about a concept you're a little shaky on (or speak aloud to an imaginary audience if necessary). As you try to summarize, define, give examples, and answer your friend's questions, you'll understand the concepts better and they will stay with you longer. Finally, step back for a big picture view and ask yourself how each piece of information fits with the whole subject. When you link the different concepts together and see them working together as a whole, it's easier to remember the individual components.

Finally, practice showing your work on any multi-step problems, even if you're just studying. Writing out each step you take to solve a problem will help solidify the process in your mind, and you'll be more likely to remember it during the test.

Modality

Modality simply refers to the means or method by which you study. Choosing a study modality that fits your own individual learning style is crucial. No two people learn best in exactly the same way, so it's important to know your strengths and use them to your advantage.

For example, if you learn best by visualization, focus on visualizing a concept in your mind and draw an image or a diagram. Try color-coding your notes, illustrating them, or creating symbols that will trigger your mind to recall a learned concept. If you learn best by hearing or discussing information, find a study partner who learns the same way or read aloud to yourself. Think about how to put the information in your own words. Imagine that you are giving a lecture on the topic and record yourself so you can listen to it later.

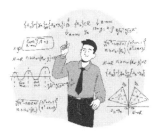

For any learning style, flashcards can be helpful. Organize the information so you can take advantage of spare moments to review. Underline key words or phrases. Use different colors for different categories. Mnemonic devices (such as creating a short list in which every item starts with the same letter) can also help with retention. Find what works best for you and use it to store the information in your mind most effectively and easily.

3

Secret Key #3 – Practice the Right Way

Your success on test day depends not only on how many hours you put into preparing, but also on whether you prepared the right way. It's good to check along the way to see if your studying is paying off. One of the most effective ways to do this is by taking practice tests to evaluate your progress. Practice tests are useful because they show exactly where you need to improve. Every time you take a practice test, pay special attention to these three groups of questions:

- The questions you got wrong
- The questions you had to guess on, even if you guessed right
- The questions you found difficult or slow to work through

This will show you exactly what your weak areas are, and where you need to devote more study time. Ask yourself why each of these questions gave you trouble. Was it because you didn't understand the material? Was it because you didn't remember the vocabulary? Do you need more repetitions on this type of question to build speed and confidence? Dig into those questions and figure out how you can strengthen your weak areas as you go back to review the material.

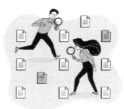 Additionally, many practice tests have a section explaining the answer choices. It can be tempting to read the explanation and think that you now have a good understanding of the concept. However, an explanation likely only covers part of the question's broader context. Even if the explanation makes perfect sense, **go back and investigate** every concept related to the question until you're positive you have a thorough understanding.

As you go along, keep in mind that the practice test is just that: practice. Memorizing these questions and answers will not be very helpful on the actual test because it is unlikely to have any of the same exact questions. If you only know the right answers to the sample questions, you won't be prepared for the real thing. **Study the concepts** until you understand them fully, and then you'll be able to answer any question that shows up on the test.

It's important to wait on the practice tests until you're ready. If you take a test on your first day of study, you may be overwhelmed by the amount of material covered and how much you need to learn. Work up to it gradually.

On test day, you'll need to be prepared for answering questions, managing your time, and using the test-taking strategies you've learned. It's a lot to balance, like a mental marathon that will have a big impact on your future. Like training for a marathon, you'll need to start slowly and work your way up. When test day arrives, you'll be ready.

Start with the strategies you've read in the first two Secret Keys—plan your course and study in the way that works best for you. If you have time, consider using multiple study resources to get different approaches to the same concepts. It can be helpful to see difficult concepts from more than one angle. Then find a good source for practice tests. Many times, the test website will suggest potential study resources or provide sample tests.

Practice Test Strategy

If you're able to find at least three practice tests, we recommend this strategy:

UNTIMED AND OPEN-BOOK PRACTICE

Take the first test with no time constraints and with your notes and study guide handy. Take your time and focus on applying the strategies you've learned.

TIMED AND OPEN-BOOK PRACTICE

Take the second practice test open-book as well, but set a timer and practice pacing yourself to finish in time.

TIMED AND CLOSED-BOOK PRACTICE

Take any other practice tests as if it were test day. Set a timer and put away your study materials. Sit at a table or desk in a quiet room, imagine yourself at the testing center, and answer questions as quickly and accurately as possible.

Keep repeating timed and closed-book tests on a regular basis until you run out of practice tests or it's time for the actual test. Your mind will be ready for the schedule and stress of test day, and you'll be able to focus on recalling the material you've learned.

Secret Key #4 – Pace Yourself

Once you're fully prepared for the material on the test, your biggest challenge on test day will be managing your time. Just knowing that the clock is ticking can make you panic even if you have plenty of time left. Work on pacing yourself so you can build confidence against the time constraints of the exam. Pacing is a difficult skill to master, especially in a high-pressure environment, so **practice is vital**.

Set time expectations for your pace based on how much time is available. For example, if a section has 60 questions and the time limit is 30 minutes, you know you have to average 30 seconds or less per question in order to answer them all. Although 30 seconds is the hard limit, set 25 seconds per question as your goal, so you reserve extra time to spend on harder questions. When you budget extra time for the harder questions, you no longer have any reason to stress when those questions take longer to answer.

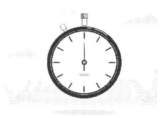

Don't let this time expectation distract you from working through the test at a calm, steady pace, but keep it in mind so you don't spend too much time on any one question. Recognize that taking extra time on one question you don't understand may keep you from answering two that you do understand later in the test. If your time limit for a question is up and you're still not sure of the answer, mark it and move on, and come back to it later if the time and the test format allow. If the testing format doesn't allow you to return to earlier questions, just make an educated guess; then put it out of your mind and move on.

On the easier questions, be careful not to rush. It may seem wise to hurry through them so you have more time for the challenging ones, but it's not worth missing one if you know the concept and just didn't take the time to read the question fully. Work efficiently but make sure you understand the question and have looked at all of the answer choices, since more than one may seem right at first.

Even if you're paying attention to the time, you may find yourself a little behind at some point. You should speed up to get back on track, but do so wisely. Don't panic; just take a few seconds less on each question until you're caught up. Don't guess without thinking, but do look through the answer choices and eliminate any you know are wrong. If you can get down to two choices, it is often worthwhile to guess from those. Once you've chosen an answer, move on and don't dwell on any that you skipped or had to hurry through. If a question was taking too long, chances are it was one of the harder ones, so you weren't as likely to get it right anyway.

On the other hand, if you find yourself getting ahead of schedule, it may be beneficial to slow down a little. The more quickly you work, the more likely you are to make a careless mistake that will affect your score. You've budgeted time for each question, so don't be afraid to spend that time. Practice an efficient but careful pace to get the most out of the time you have.

Secret Key #5 – Have a Plan for Guessing

When you're taking the test, you may find yourself stuck on a question. Some of the answer choices seem better than others, but you don't see the one answer choice that is obviously correct. What do you do?

The scenario described above is very common, yet most test takers have not effectively prepared for it. Developing and practicing a plan for guessing may be one of the single most effective uses of your time as you get ready for the exam.

In developing your plan for guessing, there are three questions to address:

- When should you start the guessing process?
- How should you narrow down the choices?
- Which answer should you choose?

When to Start the Guessing Process

Unless your plan for guessing is to select C every time (which, despite its merits, is not what we recommend), you need to leave yourself enough time to apply your answer elimination strategies. Since you have a limited amount of time for each question, that means that if you're going to give yourself the best shot at guessing correctly, you have to decide quickly whether or not you will guess.

Of course, the best-case scenario is that you don't have to guess at all, so first, see if you can answer the question based on your knowledge of the subject and basic reasoning skills. Focus on the key words in the question and try to jog your memory of related topics. Give yourself a chance to bring the knowledge to mind, but once you realize that you don't have (or you can't access) the knowledge you need to answer the question, it's time to start the guessing process.

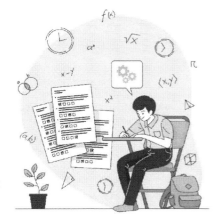

It's almost always better to start the guessing process too early than too late. It only takes a few seconds to remember something and answer the question from knowledge. Carefully eliminating wrong answer choices takes longer. Plus, going through the process of eliminating answer choices can actually help jog your memory.

Summary: Start the guessing process as soon as you decide that you can't answer the question based on your knowledge.

How to Narrow Down the Choices

The next chapter in this book (**Test-Taking Strategies**) includes a wide range of strategies for how to approach questions and how to look for answer choices to eliminate. You will definitely want to read those carefully, practice them, and figure out which ones work best for you. Here though, we're going to address a mindset rather than a particular strategy.

Your odds of guessing an answer correctly depend on how many options you are choosing from.

Number of options left	5	4	3	2	1
Odds of guessing correctly	20%	25%	33%	50%	100%

You can see from this chart just how valuable it is to be able to eliminate incorrect answers and make an educated guess, but there are two things that many test takers do that cause them to miss out on the benefits of guessing:

- Accidentally eliminating the correct answer
- Selecting an answer based on an impression

We'll look at the first one here, and the second one in the next section.

To avoid accidentally eliminating the correct answer, we recommend a thought exercise called **the $5 challenge**. In this challenge, you only eliminate an answer choice from contention if you are willing to bet $5 on it being wrong. Why $5? Five dollars is a small but not insignificant amount of money. It's an amount you could afford to lose but wouldn't want to throw away. And while losing

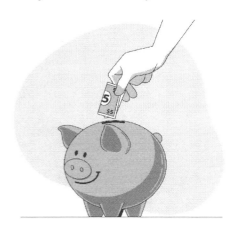

$5 once might not hurt too much, doing it twenty times will set you back $100. In the same way, each small decision you make—eliminating a choice here, guessing on a question there—won't by itself impact your score very much, but when you put them all together, they can make a big difference. By holding each answer choice elimination decision to a higher standard, you can reduce the risk of accidentally eliminating the correct answer.

The $5 challenge can also be applied in a positive sense: If you are willing to bet $5 that an answer choice *is* correct, go ahead and mark it as correct.

Summary: Only eliminate an answer choice if you are willing to bet $5 that it is wrong.

8

Which Answer to Choose

You're taking the test. You've run into a hard question and decided you'll have to guess. You've eliminated all the answer choices you're willing to bet $5 on. Now you have to pick an answer. Why do we even need to talk about this? Why can't you just pick whichever one you feel like when the time comes?

The answer to these questions is that if you don't come into the test with a plan, you'll rely on your impression to select an answer choice, and if you do that, you risk falling into a trap. The test writers know that everyone who takes their test will be guessing on some of the questions, so they intentionally write wrong answer choices to seem plausible. You still have to pick an answer though, and if the wrong answer choices are designed to look right, how can you ever be sure that you're not falling for their trap? The best solution we've found to this dilemma is to take the decision out of your hands entirely. Here is the process we recommend:

Once you've eliminated any choices that you are confident (willing to bet $5) are wrong, select the first remaining choice as your answer.

Whether you choose to select the first remaining choice, the second, or the last, the important thing is that you use some preselected standard. Using this approach guarantees that you will not be enticed into selecting an answer choice that looks right, because you are not basing your decision on how the answer choices look.

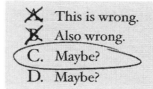

This is not meant to make you question your knowledge. Instead, it is to help you recognize the difference between your knowledge and your impressions. There's a huge difference between thinking an answer is right because of what you know, and thinking an answer is right because it looks or sounds like it should be right.

Summary: To ensure that your selection is appropriately random, make a predetermined selection from among all answer choices you have not eliminated.

Test-Taking Strategies

This section contains a list of test-taking strategies that you may find helpful as you work through the test. By taking what you know and applying logical thought, you can maximize your chances of answering any question correctly!

It is very important to realize that every question is different and every person is different: no single strategy will work on every question, and no single strategy will work for every person. That's why we've included all of them here, so you can try them out and determine which ones work best for different types of questions and which ones work best for you.

Question Strategies

☑ READ CAREFULLY

Read the question and the answer choices carefully. Don't miss the question because you misread the terms. You have plenty of time to read each question thoroughly and make sure you understand what is being asked. Yet a happy medium must be attained, so don't waste too much time. You must read carefully and efficiently.

☑ CONTEXTUAL CLUES

Look for contextual clues. If the question includes a word you are not familiar with, look at the immediate context for some indication of what the word might mean. Contextual clues can often give you all the information you need to decipher the meaning of an unfamiliar word. Even if you can't determine the meaning, you may be able to narrow down the possibilities enough to make a solid guess at the answer to the question.

☑ PREFIXES

If you're having trouble with a word in the question or answer choices, try dissecting it. Take advantage of every clue that the word might include. Prefixes can be a huge help. Usually, they allow you to determine a basic meaning. *Pre-* means before, *post-* means after, *pro-* is positive, *de-* is negative. From prefixes, you can get an idea of the general meaning of the word and try to put it into context.

☑ HEDGE WORDS

Watch out for critical hedge words, such as *likely, may, can, sometimes, often, almost, mostly, usually, generally, rarely,* and *sometimes.* Question writers insert these hedge phrases to cover every possibility. Often an answer choice will be wrong simply because it leaves no room for exception. Be on guard for answer choices that have definitive words such as *exactly* and *always.*

☑ SWITCHBACK WORDS

Stay alert for *switchbacks.* These are the words and phrases frequently used to alert you to shifts in thought. The most common switchback words are *but, although,* and *however.* Others include *nevertheless, on the other hand, even though, while, in spite of, despite,* and *regardless of.* Switchback words are important to catch because they can change the direction of the question or an answer choice.

10

⊘ Face Value

When in doubt, use common sense. Accept the situation in the problem at face value. Don't read too much into it. These problems will not require you to make wild assumptions. If you have to go beyond creativity and warp time or space in order to have an answer choice fit the question, then you should move on and consider the other answer choices. These are normal problems rooted in reality. The applicable relationship or explanation may not be readily apparent, but it is there for you to figure out. Use your common sense to interpret anything that isn't clear.

Answer Choice Strategies

⊘ Answer Selection

The most thorough way to pick an answer choice is to identify and eliminate wrong answers until only one is left, then confirm it is the correct answer. Sometimes an answer choice may immediately seem right, but be careful. The test writers will usually put more than one reasonable answer choice on each question, so take a second to read all of them and make sure that the other choices are not equally obvious. As long as you have time left, it is better to read every answer choice than to pick the first one that looks right without checking the others.

⊘ Answer Choice Families

An answer choice family consists of two (in rare cases, three) answer choices that are very similar in construction and cannot all be true at the same time. If you see two answer choices that are direct opposites or parallels, one of them is usually the correct answer. For instance, if one answer choice says that quantity x increases and another either says that quantity x decreases (opposite) or says that quantity y increases (parallel), then those answer choices would fall into the same family. An answer choice that doesn't match the construction of the answer choice family is more likely to be incorrect. Most questions will not have answer choice families, but when they do appear, you should be prepared to recognize them.

⊘ Eliminate Answers

Eliminate answer choices as soon as you realize they are wrong, but make sure you consider all possibilities. If you are eliminating answer choices and realize that the last one you are left with is also wrong, don't panic. Start over and consider each choice again. There may be something you missed the first time that you will realize on the second pass.

⊘ Avoid Fact Traps

Don't be distracted by an answer choice that is factually true but doesn't answer the question. You are looking for the choice that answers the question. Stay focused on what the question is asking for so you don't accidentally pick an answer that is true but incorrect. Always go back to the question and make sure the answer choice you've selected actually answers the question and is not merely a true statement.

⊘ Extreme Statements

In general, you should avoid answers that put forth extreme actions as standard practice or proclaim controversial ideas as established fact. An answer choice that states the "process should be used in certain situations, if..." is much more likely to be correct than one that states the "process should be discontinued completely." The first is a calm rational statement and doesn't even make a definitive, uncompromising stance, using a hedge word *if* to provide wiggle room, whereas the second choice is far more extreme.

11

⊘ Benchmark

As you read through the answer choices and you come across one that seems to answer the question well, mentally select that answer choice. This is not your final answer, but it's the one that will help you evaluate the other answer choices. The one that you selected is your benchmark or standard for judging each of the other answer choices. Every other answer choice must be compared to your benchmark. That choice is correct until proven otherwise by another answer choice beating it. If you find a better answer, then that one becomes your new benchmark. Once you've decided that no other choice answers the question as well as your benchmark, you have your final answer.

⊘ Predict the Answer

Before you even start looking at the answer choices, it is often best to try to predict the answer. When you come up with the answer on your own, it is easier to avoid distractions and traps because you will know exactly what to look for. The right answer choice is unlikely to be word-for-word what you came up with, but it should be a close match. Even if you are confident that you have the right answer, you should still take the time to read each option before moving on.

General Strategies

⊘ Tough Questions

If you are stumped on a problem or it appears too hard or too difficult, don't waste time. Move on! Remember though, if you can quickly check for obviously incorrect answer choices, your chances of guessing correctly are greatly improved. Before you completely give up, at least try to knock out a couple of possible answers. Eliminate what you can and then guess at the remaining answer choices before moving on.

⊘ Check Your Work

Since you will probably not know every term listed and the answer to every question, it is important that you get credit for the ones that you do know. Don't miss any questions through careless mistakes. If at all possible, try to take a second to look back over your answer selection and make sure you've selected the correct answer choice and haven't made a costly careless mistake (such as marking an answer choice that you didn't mean to mark). This quick double check should more than pay for itself in caught mistakes for the time it costs.

⊘ Pace Yourself

It's easy to be overwhelmed when you're looking at a page full of questions; your mind is confused and full of random thoughts, and the clock is ticking down faster than you would like. Calm down and maintain the pace that you have set for yourself. Especially as you get down to the last few minutes of the test, don't let the small numbers on the clock make you panic. As long as you are on track by monitoring your pace, you are guaranteed to have time for each question.

⊘ Don't Rush

It is very easy to make errors when you are in a hurry. Maintaining a fast pace in answering questions is pointless if it makes you miss questions that you would have gotten right otherwise. Test writers like to include distracting information and wrong answers that seem right. Taking a little extra time to avoid careless mistakes can make all the difference in your test score. Find a pace that allows you to be confident in the answers that you select.

⊘ KEEP MOVING

Panicking will not help you pass the test, so do your best to stay calm and keep moving. Taking deep breaths and going through the answer elimination steps you practiced can help to break through a stress barrier and keep your pace.

Final Notes

The combination of a solid foundation of content knowledge and the confidence that comes from practicing your plan for applying that knowledge is the key to maximizing your performance on test day. As your foundation of content knowledge is built up and strengthened, you'll find that the strategies included in this chapter become more and more effective in helping you quickly sift through the distractions and traps of the test to isolate the correct answer.

Now that you're preparing to move forward into the test content chapters of this book, be sure to keep your goal in mind. As you read, think about how you will be able to apply this information on the test. If you've already seen sample questions for the test and you have an idea of the question format and style, try to come up with questions of your own that you can answer based on what you're reading. This will give you valuable practice applying your knowledge in the same ways you can expect to on test day.

Good luck and good studying!

Physical Care Skills

Hygiene

A.M. AND H.S. CARE

A.M. (morning) care is typically done in the morning, prior to any scheduled medical procedures. A.M. care involves a complete bath, shaving, dressing, hair care, oral care, and nail care, and may require changing of the bed linens.

H.S. (hour of sleep) care is done at bedtime. H.S. care involves an abbreviated form of skin care, including washing the patient's face and hands. Oral care should also be performed. A back rub may be given for 5-10 minutes to ensure the patient is relaxed and ready for sleep. Additional tasks may be performed, depending upon the patient's level of health and activity.

HAIR CARE

Hair care is a procedure that helps to improve patient comfort and morale. It stimulates blood circulation within the scalp. Hair washing also removes excess oils and bacteria. Frequency of hair care depends upon the amount of oil that has accumulated in the patient's hair, as well as the level of dryness of the scalp.

The nurse aide must be vigilant while performing hair care. Head lice, an excessive amount of dandruff, or sores on the scalp should be **reported to the nurse immediately** if noticed by the nurse aide. Such findings may require special precautions to be taken while performing hair care in the future.

PROCEDURE FOR PERFORMING HAIR CARE

The procedure for performing hair care is as follows:

1. Raise the head of the bed to a comfortable level and place a towel beneath the patient's head.
2. Part the patient's hair into manageable sections, and run the comb or brush slowly through it. If the hair is tangled, hold the strand of hair above the tangle while combing it to prevent pulling the patient's hair.
3. While combing, carefully inspect the scalp for any lesions, lice, or signs of dryness.
4. Try to shape the hair into the patient's preferred style; even parting the hair on the correct side can provide a greater level of comfort for the patient.
5. After hair care is complete, remove the towel and reposition the patient for comfort.

NAIL CARE

Nail care is important for a number of reasons. The primary purpose of nail care is to remove bacteria and dirt from the patient's nail beds, preventing the spread of microorganisms. Appropriate nail care also ensures the patient's nails are not sharp or jagged, which increases the risk of infection from breakage of the skin. While performing nail care, the nurse aide has the opportunity to inspect the patient's nail beds for any signs of inflammation or fungal growth. Any signs of infection or discoloration should immediately be reported to the nurse.

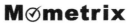

EXERCISING CAUTION DURING NAIL CARE

Prior to performing nail care, the nurse aide should check the facility policies to ensure that nail cutting falls within their scope of practice. A nurse aide should **exercise caution** when providing nail care to specific patients:

- **Patients who are receiving anticoagulation therapy**: This type of medication puts the patient at an increased risk for bleeding.
- **Patients with diabetes or peripheral vascular disease that decreases circulation to the feet**: Nail care should not be performed on these patients by the nurse aide, as these patients require foot care be performed by a professional. Diabetes and low circulation affect the ability of the tissue to repair itself. As a result, even the smallest cut on the skin places the patient at risk for severe ulcers on the feet.

PROCEDURE FOR PROPER NAIL CARE

The procedure for proper nail care is as follows:

1. Soak the patient's hands and feet in warm water to soften them and prevent the nails from cracking.
2. Carefully remove any dirt from beneath the patient's nails.
3. Trim each nail by cutting straight across with a pair of nail clippers, then round the edges using an emery board. Be careful not to cut the nails too short as this may cause irritation to the nail bed.
4. If desired, apply lotion to the patient's nails.
5. After nail care has been completed, reposition the patient for comfort and wash hands.

ORAL CARE

ABNORMAL FINDINGS

Performing oral care presents an ideal opportunity to examine the patient's oral mucosa for **abnormalities**. The nurse aide should carefully observe the patient's mouth for any sores, redness, or bleeding on the patient's lips or gums. Cracking may occur on the patient's lips as a result of dryness. The nurse aide should also be observant for any odor that may occur as a result of infection. Thrush is a fungal infection that can develop as a result of poor oral care or after taking certain medications. If thrush is present, the patient may appear with white patches covering the tongue or gums. The patient may also complain of a thick, furry feeling in the mouth.

UNCONSCIOUS PATIENTS

When performing oral care on the **unconscious patient**, first drape a towel over the patient's chest. Adjust the level of the bed to a comfortable height and raise the head of the bed greater than 30 degrees. Turn the patient's head toward oneself and hold the mouth open with a tongue depressor in one hand. Clean the patient's teeth, gums, and tongue. After cleaning has been completed, suction the secretions out of the patient's mouth. Position the patient for comfort, remove the gloves, and wash one's hands.

CONSCIOUS PATIENTS

Some **conscious patients** may not be able to perform oral care on themselves as a result of palsy or weakness in the upper extremities, therefore it is the responsibility of the nurse aide to assist them in this process. The following procedure should be followed:

1. After donning gloves, drape a towel over the patient.
2. Raise the level of the bed to a comfortable height, and position the head of the bed greater than 30 degrees.
3. Using a toothbrush, thoroughly clean the patient's teeth, gums, and tongue.
4. While performing oral care, carefully inspect the patient's mouth for any lesions or signs of infection.
5. If the patient is able to take small amounts of water without aspirating, allow them to rinse their mouth and spit the water into an emesis basin.
6. Position the patient for comfort and wash hands.

DENTURE CARE

Denture care is a common requirement for elderly patients. The procedure is as follows:

1. Obtain the patient's dentures, which are often kept in a specific cup if they are not already in the patient's mouth.
2. Place a towel or washcloth in the sink to prevent breakage if the dentures are accidentally dropped.
3. Using a toothbrush, clean the surface of the patient's dentures.
4. Place the dentures in a denture cup filled with cool water.
5. Provide oral care to the patient using sponge swabs and mouthwash; carefully observe for any lesions or signs of infection.
6. After the procedure has been completed, ask the patient if they would like to wear their dentures. If not, place the dentures in the denture cup and place it on the patient's bedside table.
7. Position the patient for comfort and wash hands.

BATHING

PURPOSE

Over time, irritants can build on the patient's skin, which can cause a rash or skin breakdown. These irritants can also cause itching, which may provoke the patient to scratch the skin, creating a source of infection. **Bathing** cleanses the patient's skin of these irritants. Bathing can also promote patient relaxation and increase circulation. Bathing presents an opportunity to perform a thorough assessment of the patient's skin. Any signs of breakdown or lesions should be immediately reported. Furthermore, the patient's skin should be closely monitored for dryness, as this can cause cracking of the patient's skin, an additional portal of entry for infection.

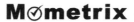

BED BATH, TUB BATH, AND PARTIAL BATH

A **tub bath** is preferred when the patient is strong enough to get into and out of the bathtub. It involves completely washing the patient, including performing perineal care. A tub bath can be given daily. However, if the patient's skin is showing signs of dryness, the frequency may be reduced to two or three times a week.

A **bed bath** is given to a patient when they are unable to ambulate. A complete bed bath involves cleansing the patient's skin and changing the patient's linens.

If the patient is incontinent of urine or stool, a **partial bath** may be given. This involves cleansing only those parts of the body that have been soiled and changing only those linens that are dirty.

NECESSARY SUPPLIES FOR A BED BATH

A bed bath can be a time-consuming procedure, depending upon the patient's level of activity. One way to facilitate a bed bath is to make sure that all of the **necessary supplies** are present prior to starting the bath. A nurse aide will require a basin of water, soap, and lotion. The water should be warmed to 105-115 °F. The nurse aide will need several washcloths and at least two towels. The nurse aide must also have a pair of gloves to wear while giving the bath. Linens should be changed while the bed bath is being performed. In order to change the bed, the nurse aide will need a fitted sheet, a bed pad, a flat sheet, a blanket, and pillowcases.

PROCEDURE FOR PERFORMING A BED BATH

The procedure for performing a **bed bath** is as follows:

1. Fill a basin with water at a temperature of 105-115 °F.
2. Remove as much medical equipment from the patient as possible.
3. Keep the patient covered to maintain dignity.
4. Allow the patient to bathe as much of himself or herself as possible.
5. Begin by washing the patient's face, moving downward to the arms, the chest, abdomen, legs, back, and perineal area.
6. Use a different washcloth for each area of the body.
7. If necessary, change the patient's bed linens while washing the back.
8. Apply lotion if desired.
9. After the bath has been completed, reposition the patient for comfort and wash hands.

PROCEDURE FOR PERFORMING TUB BATH

The procedure for performing a **tub bath** is as follows:

1. Prior to performing a tub bath, the nurse aide should sure the bathtub has been cleaned.
2. Place towels in the tub and on the floor outside the tub to prevent slipping.
3. Ambulate the patient to the tub, observing all precautions.
4. Once the patient is in the tub, fill it to the desired level. Make sure the water temperature is no greater than 115 °F.
5. Provide privacy while the patient washes, but maintain close supervision to make sure the patient does not slip.
6. Wash the patient's back and any area they are unable to reach.
7. Drain the water and dry the patient.
8. Assist the patient into a standing position and carefully help them out of the tub.
9. Assist the patient in putting on clothes.
10. Position the patient for comfort, clean the tub, and wash hands.

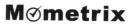

PROCEDURE FOR PROVIDING PERINEAL CARE DURING THE BATH

Perineal care is an important part of bathing because it allows the nurse aide to inspect the skin of the perineal area. If done properly, it also decreases the risk for urinary tract infections. Perineal care should be done during a complete bath and should also be performed after the patient is incontinent. The nurse aide should first wash hands and don a pair of gloves. Instruct the patient to open their legs. Cleanse the skin of the perineal area, using front to back movements. Never wash from back to front as this can introduce germs from the anus to the urethral area. After the skin has been cleansed, completely dry the area. Do not reuse the linens that were used to wash the perineal area. Obtain a clean towel and washcloth to complete the bath.

PROCEDURES TO PREVENT SKIN IRRITATION

Skin irritation can result in sores and infection. There are a number of measures a nurse aide can take to **prevent skin irritation** from occurring.

- One way to avoid skin rash or irritation is to completely **cleanse the skin of any urine or feces** if the patient has soiled himself. Because urine and stool are acidic in nature, skin breakdown can occur quickly if they are left close to the patient's skin.
- If the patient is incontinent, applying **water resistant lotion** will protect the skin by creating a barrier that will prevent rashes or breakdown.
- **Frequent repositioning** should also be performed to prevent skin breakdown. A bedridden patient should be turned every two hours to prevent breakdown over bony prominences.

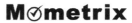

Dressing and Grooming

ADLs, Dressing, and Grooming

Activities of daily living (ADLs) are tasks that are required to keep a person healthy and functional. Often, a person's level of health is determined by their ability to perform ADLs. The tasks are divided into two subgroups:

- **Basic ADLs** are tasks people must be able to perform in order to care for themselves. These include bathing, dressing, feeding, toileting, and walking.
- **Instrumental ADLs** are tasks people must be able to perform in order to live independently within the community. These include shopping, cooking, housework, medication management, and money management.

Dressing and grooming are important basic activities of daily living, and a patient that is unable to perform these independently requires the help of the nurse aide. Prior to conducting any elements of dressing or grooming, the nurse aide must greet the patient, wash his or her own hands, and explain what is going to be done. Gloves should be worn if any risk of exposure to bodily fluid exists.

Dressing a Stroke Patient

When the patient has suffered a **stroke**, it can result in weakness on one side of the patient's body. Often, the stroke patient requires assistance in daily activities, such as dressing. It is important to teach the patient how to clothe oneself safely to promote independence and decrease the risk of falling. Before beginning to assist the patient in undressing, make sure the clean set of clothes is within easy reach. When putting on clothing, the patient should be taught to dress the weakened side of the body first, using their strong side to do so. For example, a patient with weakness on the right side should insert the right arm into the sleeve first. When removing clothes, the patient should be taught to undress the strong side first.

Shaving a Patient

If the nurse aide is to **shave a patient**, they must first apply a pair of gloves and then follow the below procedure:

1. Use a wet washcloth to moisten the hair on the patient's face and neck.
2. Check the razor to make sure it does not have any loose blades or jagged edges.
3. Drape the patient with a towel and apply shaving cream to the area that needs to be shaved.
4. Use one hand to pull the skin taut, while moving the razor with firm strokes in the direction that the hair is growing.
5. Rinse the razor in a basin of water as often as necessary.
6. Use a moistened washcloth to rinse off all remaining shaving cream.

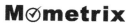

Nutrition and Hydration

NUTRIENTS

Nutrients are elements in nature that are necessary for humans to consume in order to live. Our bodies absorb the nutrients from the foods we eat. Nutrients are divided into the following groups:

- **Carbohydrates** are composed primarily of sugar and serve as the main source of energy.
- **Protein** is made primarily of amino acids and aids in tissue repair.
- **Fats** are composed of fatty acids and are essential for cell membrane integrity and thermal regulation.
- **Minerals** and **vitamins** are needed to aid metabolism and a number of other body processes.
- **Water** acts as a solvent and is also required for a number of body processes.

WATER

Water is a vitally important nutrient. It aids in metabolism, temperature regulation, and elimination of body waste. Water is constantly lost through normal sweating, elimination, and exhalation. Certain states, such as illness and increased activity, can cause increased water loss. It is recommended that the patient take in at least 1500-2000 mL or 8-10 glasses of water every day to maintain hydration and replace lost body fluids. If the patient does not receive an adequate volume of fluids, dehydration may occur. If left uncorrected, dehydration can be a fatal condition.

FEEDING PATIENTS

ASSESSING THE MEAL AND THE NEED FOR FEEDING ASSISTANCE

Before taking the tray into the patient's room, the nurse aide should check to make sure the patient is **receiving the correct tray**. Check the patient's armband and compare it to the name and room number on the tray. Check to make sure the patient's tray contains foods that are appropriate for the patient's ordered diet.

The **amount of feeding assistance** that should be provided depends upon the individual patient. Some patients will not require assistance to feed themselves. If the patient is able to feed themselves, they should be allowed to do so as a means of encouraging independence. Some assistance may be required, such as cutting larger portions and opening beverages. Some patients, such as those who suffer from blindness, may only need verbal cues to eat. Some patients are unable to feed themselves as a result of weakness or paralysis of the upper body. These patients will require their food be cut and each bite fed to them. Nurse aides should be careful to take their time and not rush the feeding. Aides should ensure the patient has chewed and swallowed every bite, before offering the next bit of food.

PROCESS FOR FEEDING A PATIENT

The process for feeding a patient is as follows:

1. Wash hands and raise the head of the patient's bed.
2. Explain to the patient what foods are being served on the tray and allow the patient to select what foods will be fed first.
3. When providing a bite to the patient, ensure the spoon is only half full. Use only the tip of the spoon to feed the patient.
4. Feed the patient slowly, ensuring the patient has swallowed all of the food in their mouth before offering the next bite.
5. Make sure the patient has had enough food to eat before taking the tray away.
6. If the patient appears to be having difficulty swallowing, stop feeding the patient immediately and notify the nurse.

CLOCK METHOD OF FEEDING PATIENTS

The clock method is a way of describing the placement of food on a plate to a visually impaired patient who is able to feed oneself. The patient should be instructed to picture the plate as a clock face, with positions of food located at corresponding numbers. For example, the meat can be at the 12 o'clock position, the vegetables at the 3 o'clock position, bread at the 6 o'clock position, and the fruit at the 9 o'clock position. The nurse aide should try to repeat this pattern at every meal so that the patient is familiar with the locations of each type of food.

TASKS PERFORMED AFTER ASSISTING THE PATIENT WITH EATING

After the patient has finished eating, remove the meal tray and calculate the amount of food the patient took in. If the patient is on a calorie count diet, calculate the percentage of food eaten and tolerance to the food. If the patient's intake and output is being monitored, calculate the amount of fluid the patient took in. Report these findings to the nurse. Position the patient for comfort and place the call light within reach. Make sure any necessary items, such as the tray table and personal items, are within reach. Hand hygiene should then be performed.

FLUID INTAKE

DEHYDRATION

Dehydration is a life-threatening condition that occurs when the body does not have enough water to perform normal body functions. Patients who are dehydrated may present with sunken eyes and dry mucous membranes. Dehydrated patients will often complain of generalized weakness and constant thirst. Their skin may lose its elasticity as a result of dehydration. They may have a weak rapid pulse and a low blood pressure. The urine will become darker and more concentrated when patients are dehydrated; a result of the kidneys conserving as much water as possible.

CAUSES OF DEHYDRATION

Dehydration can be caused by too little intake or too much output. Limited intake may result if the patient is unable to take in fluid as a result of chronic nausea or difficulty swallowing. The patient may be unable to obtain an adequate amount of fluid if they are confused or kept NPO. Dehydration may also result if the patient is excreting too much fluid. The most common cause of over-excretion of fluid is frequent diarrhea. Excessive sweating from fever or exercise may also result in excessive fluid loss. Blood loss after surgery or a hemorrhage or fluid loss after a burn may also cause dehydration.

ENCOURAGING FLUIDS

If a patient is dehydrated, they must increase the volume of fluids that they consume in order to restore fluid balance. To encourage more fluid intake, explain to the patient why it is important to consume more fluids and make sure a water pitcher and glass is within reach. Fluids should be encouraged each time the nurse aide goes into the patient's room. Also, make other fluids available, such as fruit juice or decaffeinated tea or coffee. Try to avoid sugary sodas or caffeinated beverages as these may not quench the patient's thirst. If the patient has family present, ask them to also encourage the patient to drink more.

THERAPEUTIC DIETS

NPO, CLEAR LIQUID, AND MECHANICAL SOFT

NPO (nothing by mouth) is a diet that is ordered for patients who are not allowed to eat. It is typically ordered in anticipation of medical testing or a surgical procedure. Patient status will also be made NPO if it is unsafe for the individual to eat, such as a patient who is intubated, sedated, or unable to swallow properly.

A **clear liquid** diet is the first diet prescribed after a patient is taken off NPO status. It is typically ordered to allow the patient to eat without experiencing nausea.

A **mechanical soft diet** is prescribed for patients who have difficulty chewing, such as patients who do not have their dentures. It is also intended to help patients to transition from NPO to a regular diet.

CONDITION-SPECIFIC DIETS

The diet that is prescribed for a patient depends upon the individual's health history and current diagnosis:

- A **regular diet** has no dietary restrictions; patients can eat whatever they like.
- A **calorie count diet** is typically ordered for diabetic patients; it limits the amount of sugar the patient takes in and counts the number of calories and carbohydrates the patient consumes.
- A **low-sodium diet** is prescribed to limit the amount of salt ingested by patients with a history of renal impairment or hypertension.
- A **cardiac diet** is ordered for patients with a history of cardiac problems; while on this diet, they are served low-fat, low-calorie, and low-sodium foods.

ASPIRATION

INDICATIONS

A helpless patient is at a significant risk for aspirating food. During **aspiration**, small amounts of food and water move down the trachea and into the patient's lungs. Forceful coughing or a wet-sounding voice after swallowing a bite of food may be an indication of aspiration. If a patient needs to chew food for long periods of time or requires multiple attempts to swallow food, they may be aspirating. Other indications include unusual head movements while trying to swallow, difficulty breathing, drooling while eating, or pocketing food in the cheeks. All of these signs should be reported to the patient's nurse.

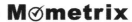

ASPIRATION PRECAUTIONS

Aspiration precautions are steps that are taken when a patient has difficulty swallowing to prevent food and drink from going into the lungs. Prior to being fed, the patient should be positioned with the head of the bed at a 90° angle. The nurse aide should check to make sure the patient's food and drink is thickened to the prescribed consistency. The patient should be fed slowly, with the nurse aide offering small amounts of food on a spoon. The patient should be allowed an adequate amount of time to chew and swallow. After the meal has been completed, the patient should remain upright for at least a half-hour to prevent reflux. After a half-hour has passed, the patient can be repositioned for comfort.

MEETING PATIENT'S PERSONAL DIETARY NEEDS

Upon admission to the hospital or long-term care facility, the nurse aide should make note of any cultural or religious requests that the patient may have regarding **personal dietary needs**. The facility dietary service should be notified as soon as possible to ensure the patient is provided with appropriate foods. Prior to taking the tray in to the room, the nurse aide should check to make sure the food on the tray meets the patient's dietary restrictions. If it does not, the dietary service should be notified regarding the problem, and a replacement meal should be obtained as soon as possible.

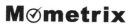

Elimination

INDWELLING CATHETERS

An **indwelling or Foley catheter** is typically placed in patients that are unable to completely empty their bladder while voiding or are on sedation that makes them unable to control urination. It is also placed in patients with chronic issues of the bladder. It may also be placed for incontinent and immobile patients to protect their skin from the acidity of the urine. Post-surgical or critical care patients may receive an indwelling catheter in order to accurately measure their urinary output. The indwelling catheter is placed by a nurse (with some facilities requiring a second nurse be present) using sterile technique. A latex or silicone catheter is inserted into the patient's urethra and into the bladder. A bulb at the end of the tube is inflated using sterile water, which keeps the tube in place and prevents leakage around the catheter. An indwelling catheter places the patient at an increased risk of developing a urinary tract infection, therefore catheter care should be performed frequently, and the catheter should be removed as soon as possible.

FINDINGS TO REPORT

When a patient has an indwelling catheter, the nurse aide should **report** the following:

- The **amount of urine drained** from the catheter should be noted and reported to the patient's nurse. If the patient is not urinating enough (less than 30 mL per hour) or too much without the administration of a diuretic (greater than 400 mL per hour), the nurse should be notified.
- The **appearance** of the urine should also be monitored, and any abnormalities should be reported. Abnormal findings include cloudiness, sediment in the urine, or an unusual color, such as dark amber or green. The nurse should also be notified if the patient's urine is blood-tinged or foul smelling.
- The nurse should be notified if the **patient complains of pain or fullness in the bladder** as this may indicate that the catheter has clotted and requires irrigation.

PLACING PATIENT ON BEDPAN

When a patient without an indwelling catheter is bedbound and requests to use the bathroom, a bedpan should be provided. The nurse aide should follow the below procedures **when placing a patient on the bedpan**:

1. Wash hands and greet the patient. Explain what is going to be done.
2. Make sure the patient has privacy by drawing the curtain and don a pair of gloves.
3. Lay the patient in a supine (flat) position and then turn them on their side.
4. Place the bedpan over the buttocks and carefully roll the patient back onto their back. Some patients may benefit from having an absorbent pad placed over the bed pan prior to positioning it in order to prevent leakage.
5. Instruct the patient to open their legs and ensure the bedpan has been placed properly.
6. Raise the head of the bed to the patient's requested position, give the patient the call bell, and instruct the patient to call when finished.
7. Remove the gloves and wash hands.
8. Provide privacy by drawing the curtain or closing the door upon exiting.

GETTING PATIENT OFF OF BEDPAN

When the patient is ready to get **off the bedpan,** the nurse aide should do as follows:

1. Ensure patient privacy.
2. Wash hands and don a pair of gloves.
3. Lay the head of the bed flat and turn the patient on their side.
4. While turning the patient, support the bedpan in order to prevent secretions from leaking into the bed.
5. Remove the bedpan and set it to one side.
6. Provide perineal care for the patient.
7. Position the patient for comfort and allow them to wash their hands with a damp rag or wipe, if desired.
8. Measure the output and dispose of the secretions.

ABNORMAL BOWEL MOVEMENTS

There are various abnormalities in bowel movements that the nurse aide should be aware of when caring for their patients. Symptoms of any of the following should be reported to the nurse:

- **Constipation** occurs when the patient's stool is too dry and hard to be able to be passed easily, making the patient unable to have a bowel movement. The feces become dry and hard as a result of too much water being absorbed from the stool due to poor gastrointestinal motility. If the constipation is not treated, the patient may develop a bowel obstruction.
- **Diarrhea** refers to the frequent passage of loose or watery stools. Diarrhea places the patient at risk for developing dehydration because of the amount of fluid lost with the stool. Electrolytes are passed along with the fluid, which can lead to life-threatening electrolyte imbalances if not properly corrected.
- **Gastrointestinal (GI) bleeding** can be a dangerous complication for patients and signs should be immediately reported to the nurse. GI bleeds that originate in the upper GI tract produce dark, tarry stools. GI bleeds that originate in the lower GI tract produce frank (bright red) blood in the stool. Observations of either of these color changes must be immediately reported to the nurse. The nurse aide should remain with the patient if they are showing any symptoms of hypotension (mental status changes, rapid pulse or respiratory rate, lowered blood pressure) that could indicate GI hemorrhage (life-threatening bleeding).

CARING FOR PATIENT WHO IS CONSTIPATED

During hospitalization, there is a strong risk that the patient will develop constipation. This is often the result of decreased activity and the administration of medications that reduce gastrointestinal motility (most commonly, narcotics). The patient's bowel habits should be closely monitored. If the patient is using a bedpan, the consistency, color, and amount of stool should be noted after every bowel movement. If the patient is able to go to the bathroom without assistance, the nurse aide should inquire about the quality and frequency of the patient's stools. Some patients may be advised not to flush after using the toilet so that these qualities can be directly observed by the nurse aide. If the patient is constipated, it is important to encourage fluids to prevent drying of the stool. Warm liquids and juices are particularly effective in improving gastrointestinal motility. Foods that are high in fiber should also be encouraged. Caffeinated beverages should be avoided.

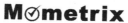

CARING FOR PATIENT WITH DIARRHEA

Patients who experience multiple bouts of diarrhea should be closely monitored for any signs or symptoms of dehydration. The number of stools and amount of fluid that are passed should be monitored. A stool specimen should be collected as soon as possible to determine the cause of the diarrhea. If the patient is having frequent diarrhea, it is important to encourage them to drink fluids to prevent them from becoming dehydrated. If their diet allows, the patient should be encouraged to drink two glasses of fluid for every bout of diarrhea. Proper hand hygiene should also be encouraged.

URINARY TRACT INFECTION
SIGNS AND SYMPTOMS

The **primary symptom** of a urinary tract infection is painful or difficult urination. The patient may exhibit cloudy urine, which may have a strong or foul smell. The patient may experience the need to urinate frequently or may have sudden urgency in the need to urinate. The patient may also complain of flank pain or pressure in the pelvis. The patient may show signs of a generalized infection, such as an elevated temperature, flushed skin, or malaise. An elderly patient may also show signs of confusion as a result of the infection.

PREVENTION

There are a number of ways that a urinary tract infection can be **prevented**. If a patient's diet tolerates it, oral fluids should be encouraged. Cranberry juice is particularly helpful in preventing urinary tract infections because it raises the acidity of the urine. If the patient needs assistance to void, help them to the bathroom as soon as possible, as holding in urine can increase the patient's risk for developing an infection. While performing perineal care, the nurse aide should make sure to wash female patients from front to back. If the patient is able to ambulate, showers should be encouraged rather than baths.

BLADDER TRAINING

Bladder training usually requires the person to keep a toileting diary for at least three days so patterns can be assessed. There are a number of different approaches:

- **Scheduled toileting** is toileting on a regular schedule, usually every 2-4 hours during the daytime.
- **Habit training** involves an attempt to match the scheduled toileting to a person's individual voiding habits, based on the toileting diary. This is useful for people who have a natural and fairly consistent voiding pattern. Toileting is done every 2-4 hours.
- **Prompted voiding** is often used in nursing homes and attempts to teach people to assess their own incontinence status and prompts them to ask for toileting.
- **Bladder retraining** is a behavioral modification program that teaches people to inhibit the urge to urinate and to urinate according to an established schedule, restoring normal bladder function as much as possible. Bladder training can improve incontinence in 80% of cases.

PROMPTED VOIDING

Prompted voiding is a communication protocol for people with mild to moderate **cognitive impairment**. It uses positive reinforcement for recognizing being wet or dry, staying dry, urinating, and drinking liquids.

- Ask patient **every two hours** (8 a.m. to 4-8 p.m.) whether they are wet or dry.
- Verify if they are correct and give **feedback**, "You are right, Mrs. Brown, you are dry."

27

- **Prompt** patient, whether wet or dry, to use the toilet or urinal. If yes, assist them, record results, and give positive reinforcement by praising and visiting for a short time. If no, repeat the request again once or twice. If they are wet, and decline toileting, change and tell them you will return in two hours and ask them to try to wait to urinate until then.
- Offer **liquids** and record amount.
- **Record** results of each attempt to urinate or wet check.

BLADDER RETRAINING

Bladder retraining teaches people to control the urge to urinate. It usually takes about three months to rehabilitate a bladder muscle weakened from frequent urination, causing a decreased urinary capacity. A short urination interval is gradually lengthened to every 2-4 hours during the daytime as the person suppresses bladder urges and stays dry.

- The patient keeps a **urination diary** for a week.
- An individual program is established with **scheduled voiding times and goals**. For example, if a patient is urinating every hour, the goal might be every 80 minutes with increased output.
- The patient is taught **techniques** to withhold urination, such as sitting on a hard seat or on a tightly rolled towel to put pressure on pelvic floor muscles, doing five squeezes of pelvic floor muscles, deep breathing, and counting backward from 50.
- When the patient consistently meets the goal, a **new goal** is established.

THE KNACK TO CONTROL URINARY INCONTINENCE

The **knack** is the use of precisely timed muscle contractions to prevent **stress incontinence**. It is "the knack" of squeezing up before bearing down. The knack is a preventive use of **Kegel exercises**. Women are taught to contract the pelvic floor muscles right before and during events that usually cause stress incontinence. For example, if a woman feels a cough or sneeze coming, she immediately contracts the pelvic floor muscles and holds until the stress event is over. This contraction augments support of the proximal urethra, reducing the amount of displacement that usually takes place with compromised muscle support, thereby preventing incontinence. It is particularly useful if used before and during stress events, such as coughing, sneezing, lifting, standing, swinging a golf club, or laughing. Studies have shown that women who are taught this technique for mild to moderate urinary incontinence and use it consistently are able to decrease incontinence by 73-98%.

BOWEL TRAINING

Bowel training for defecation includes keeping a bowel diary to chart progress:

- **Scheduled defecation** is usually daily, but for some people 3-4 times weekly, depending on individual bowel habits. Defecation should be at the same time, so work hours and activities must be considered. Defecation is scheduled for 20-30 minutes after a meal when there is increased motility.
- **Stimulation** is necessary. Drinking a cup of hot liquid may work, but initially many require rectal stimulation, inserting a gloved, lubricated finger into the anus and running it around the rim of the sphincters. Some people require rectal suppositories, such as glycerine. Stimulus suppositories, such as Dulcolax (bisacodyl), or even Fleet enemas are sometimes used, but the goal is to reduce use of medical or chemical stimulants.
- **Position** should be sitting upright with knees elevated slightly if possible and leaning forward during defecation.

- **Straining** includes attempting to tighten abdominal muscles and relax sphincters while defecating.
- **Exercise** increases the motility of the bowel by stimulating muscle contractions. **Walking** is one of the best exercises for this purpose, and the person should try to walk 1 or 2 miles a day. If the person is unable to walk, then other activities, such as chair exercises that involve the arms and legs and bending can be very effective. Those who are bed bound need to turn from side to side frequently and change position.
- **Kegel exercises** increase strength of the pelvic floor muscles. Kegel exercises for urinary incontinence and fecal incontinence are essentially the same, but the person tries to pull in the muscles around the anus, as though trying to prevent the release of stool or flatus. The person should feel the muscles tightening while holding for 2 seconds and then relaxing for 2 seconds, gradually building the holding time to 10 seconds or more. Exercises should be done 4 times a day.

MANAGEMENT STRATEGIES FOR CONSTIPATION AND FECAL IMPACTION

Management strategies for constipation and impaction include:

- **Enemas** and **manual removal of impaction** may be necessary initially.
- Add **fiber** with bran, fresh/dried fruits, and whole grains, to 20-35 grams per day.
- Increase **fluids** to 64 ounces each day.
- **Exercise** program should include walking if possible, and exercises on a daily basis.
- Change in **medications** causing constipation can relieve constipation. Additionally, the use of stool softeners, such as Colace (docusate), or bulk formers, such as Metamucil (psyllium), may decrease fluid absorption and move stool through the colon more quickly. Overuse of laxatives can cause constipation.
- Careful **monitoring** of diet, fluids, and medical treatment, especially for irritable bowel syndrome.
- **Pregnancy-related constipation** may be controlled through dietary and fluid modifications and regular exercise.
- **Delayed toileting** should be avoided and bowel training regimen done to promote evacuation at the same time each day. During travel, stool softeners, increased fluid, and exercise may alleviate constipation.

PURPOSE OF FIBER IN THE DIET

Most constipation is caused by insufficient **fiber** in the diet, especially if people eat a lot of processed foods. An adequate amount of fiber is 20-30 grams daily. There are both soluble and insoluble forms of fiber, and both add bulk to the stool and are not absorbed into the body. Some foods have both types:

- **Soluble fiber** dissolves in liquids to form a gel-like substance, which is why liquids are so important in conjunction with fiber in the diet. Soluble fiber slows the movement of stool through the gastrointestinal system. Food sources include bananas, potatoes, dried beans, nuts, apples, oranges, and oatmeal.
- **Insoluble fiber** changes little with the digestive process and increases the speed of stool through the colon, so too much can result in diarrhea. Food sources of insoluble fiber include wheat bran, whole grains, seeds, skins of fruits, vegetables, and nuts.

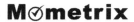

Rest, Sleep, and Comfort

MAKING AN UNOCCUPIED BED

The linens on an **unoccupied bed** can be changed easily whenever the patient is out of bed. Wash the hands and raise the level of the bed to a comfortable height. Lower all of the side rails. Don gloves and remove all of the current linens, taking care to place them in the dirty linen receptacle without letting sheets touch the body or skin (as often, dirty sheets can be soiled with bodily fluids or waste). Place the clean fitted sheet on the bed, pulling it tight to make sure it does not wrinkle. Place an absorbent pad on the bed so that it will be positioned below the patient's hips and upper legs. Carefully unfold the clean flat sheet and place it on the bed, tucking the bottom edges of the blanket tightly underneath the mattress. Place the thick blanket on the bed. Fold the top of the blanket and flat sheet back over the foot of the bed to allow the patient to enter the bed. Raise the side rails on one side of the bed, and put the bed back into the lowest position. Wash the hands.

MAKING AN OCCUPIED BED

Some patients are bedbound and therefore require new bed linens to be put on the bed while they remain in it. The patient should be informed of the process so they are not surprised or confused. Care should be taken to protect the patient's privacy by drawing the curtain and keeping the patient covered by their gown. When making an **occupied bed**, instruct or assist the patient into a lateral position (on their side) and release the dirty fitted sheet from the top and bottom corners of the side the patient is faced away from. Roll that side of the dirty fitted sheet (with the accompanying dirty absorbent pad) toward the patient, so that the side that touched the patient is inside the rolled-up linen. Next, unfold the clean fitted sheet, and place it on the half of the bed that has been unmade, tucking both the top and bottom corners firmly around the mattress. Place a new absorbent pad on the clean fitted sheet so that it will be positioned beneath the patient's hips. Roll the clean linen, and tuck it beneath the rolled dirty linen, under the patient. Slowly turn the patient over the rolled-up linen, onto the other side. Some patients may be able to do this independently, while others may require assistance or feel pain in this process, so care should be taken to assess the patient's needs. Move to the opposite side of the bed, and remove the dirty fitted sheet and pad. Place the dirty sheet and pad in the appropriate receptacle(s). Unroll the clean fitted sheet and pad, pulling it tightly to ensure there are no wrinkles. Secure the fitted sheet to the bed. Roll the patient back onto their back. Cover the patient with a new sheet and blanket and position the patient for comfort. Prior to leaving the patient's room ask if there is anything else the patient may need.

PATIENT TRANSFERS

TO THE SIDE OF THE BED

Patient strength should be assessed prior to moving the patient **to the side of the bed** to determine how much assistance may be required. While the patient is in bed, make sure the bed's brakes are locked and the bed is in the lowest position. Lower the side rail and raise the head of the bed until it is at a comfortable level for the patient. While facing the patient, place one arm behind the shoulders and one arm beneath the knees. Assist the patient into a sitting position at the side of the bed. Allow the patient to remain there for a few moments to ensure the patient is not dizzy from the change in position.

BED TO WHEELCHAIR

Care must be taken while transferring a patient **from the bed to the wheelchair** to prevent falling during the transfer. Prior to moving the patient, make sure the bed and wheelchair wheels are locked to prevent movement during ambulation. Ensure that the patient is wearing rubber-soled socks or shoes to prevent slipping and make sure the patient is not suffering from any dizziness or lightheadedness that may result from a quick change in position. Prior to beginning the transfer, explain the process to the patient.

Move the wheelchair as close to the bed as possible and make sure the wheels are locked. Lift the leg pads and footplates up and out of the way to prevent tripping. Assist the patient into a dangling position. Place the feet in a wide stance. Instruct the patient to stand on the count of three, and support the torso while helping the patient into a standing position. Pivot the patient so that their back is to the wheelchair. Instruct the patient to position their hands on the armrests of the wheelchair and back up until they feel the seat against the backs of their legs. Slowly lower the patient into a sitting position. Assist the patient in lifting their legs and placing the leg pads and footplates beneath them.

BED TO STRETCHER

While the patient is lying in bed, make sure the wheels of the bed and the **stretcher** are locked. Raise the level of the bed until it is the same height as the stretcher. If available, a slider board can be placed beneath the patient to facilitate movement and decrease friction. Stand at the side of the stretcher, and ask a colleague to stand next to the bed. Instruct the patient to cross their arms over their chest to prevent the dragging of their limbs across the bed. Grasp the draw sheet and roll it to maintain a good grip. On the count of three, pull the draw sheet toward the body, while the colleague at the side of the bed pushes the patient from the other side. Continue to pull until the patient is in the center of the stretcher. Position the patient for comfort.

AMBULATING WITH PATIENTS
LEVELS OF ASSISTANCE DURING AMBULATION

Stand by assistance (SBA), contact guard assistance (CGA), minimum assistance (MIN), and maximum assistance (MAX) refer to the **level of assistance** the patient requires while ambulating.

- A patient who can move independently requires **SBA**. This patient does not require any assistance in ambulating and does not require a gait belt.
- **CGA** refers to a patient who does not require assistance but is at risk for falling. The nursing aide should be close enough to touch the patient in case they should fall, but does not provide additional support.
- **MIN** assistance refers to the patient who needs a small amount of support while ambulating. A gait belt is advised for this type of patient.
- Patients who require **MAX** assistance may or may not be able to bear their own weight. This type of patient requires support from one or two staff members to ensure that they do not fall.

ENSURING SAFETY DURING AMBULATION

While the patient is **ambulating**, make sure to provide support using a gait belt. Ensure the patient is wearing rubber-soled slippers. If the patient is receiving oxygen therapy, obtain a rolling tank so the patient can continue to wear oxygen while ambulating. Carefully monitor the patient's respirations and frequently check to make sure the patient is not becoming fatigued or dizzy. Move at a pace that is comfortable for the patient and do not try to rush them. If necessary, allow the patient to stop to take a brief rest in a chair to ensure that they do not become overexerted.

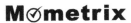

CRUTCH WALKING
PROPER FIT OF CRUTCH

Though it is the job of the physical therapist to adjust crutches properly to the size of the patient, the crutch should be checked prior to each ambulation to make sure it continues to fit properly. The pads of the crutch should remain one to one-and-a-half inches below the axillary area. The handgrips should be even with the patient's hips. When the patient is in a standing position with hands resting on the handgrips, the elbows should be slightly flexed. When the patient walks on crutches, they should support their weight with hands on the handgrips. Placing weight on the pads in the axillary area may cause nerve damage. The patient should keep the head and shoulders erect to limit back strain and keep the torso aligned with the crutches to prevent loss of balance and injury.

FOUR-POINT TECHNIQUE AND THREE-POINT TECHNIQUE

The **four-point technique** is the preferred method of ambulation for a patient with poor lower body strength who is ambulating with crutches. While the patient is standing, instruct them to move the left crutch forward first, followed by the right foot. The right crutch should then be moved forward, followed by the left foot. The advantage of this method of ambulation is that the patient has at least three points of contact with the ground at all times, offering the most stability; the disadvantage is that it requires a slow movement speed.

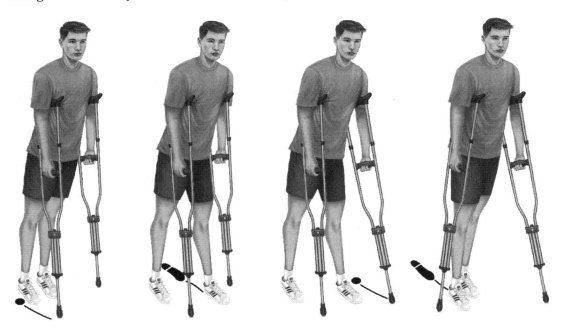

The **three-point technique** is recommended for patients who are unable to bear weight on one foot while ambulating with crutches. While in a standing position, the patient should move both crutches and the affected limb forward. Then, while placing their weight on the crutches, the patient should move their strong leg forward until it is even with the affected extremity.

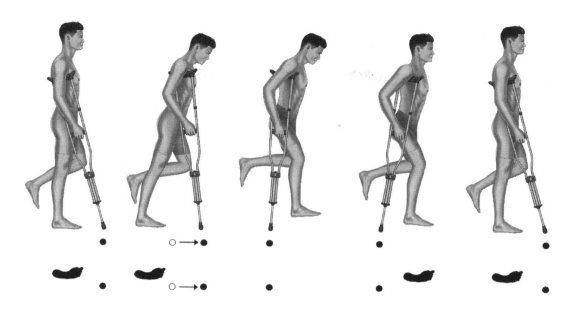

SWING-TO METHOD AND SWING-THROUGH METHOD

The **swing-to and swing-through methods of crutch walking** are intended for patients who have decreased lower body strength. Both methods are advantageous in that they are easy to learn and allow for a quick gait. The disadvantage is that both methods require strong upper body strength. In the swing-to method, both crutches are moved forward and placed at the length of a step in front of them. The patient then places their weight upon the crutches and swings their body forward until the feet are equal to the crutches. In the swing-through method, both crutches are moved forward. Placing their weight upon the crutches, the patient swings their lower body forward and places their feet slightly in front of the crutches.

TRANSFERRING PATIENT FROM CHAIR OR SITTING POSITION TO STANDING POSITION USING CRUTCHES

While the patient is sitting in the chair, instruct them to hold both crutches in one hand by gripping the handgrips. Instruct the patient to scoot their hips to the edge of the chair and stretch the non-weight-bearing foot out straight. Help the patient rise to a standing position, using the arm of the chair to support one of the patient's arms and the crutches to support the other. Once the patient has balanced their weight on one foot, instruct the patient to move one of the crutches to the opposite side and place their hands on the handgrips.

TRANSFERRING PATIENT FROM STANDING TO SITTING POSITION USING CRUTCHES

To move from a **standing to a sitting position**, instruct the patient to approach the chair until they are one step away from the front of the chair. Instruct the patient to carefully turn using their weight-bearing leg and the crutches until their back is to the chair. Assist the patient in finding their balance before transferring one of the crutches to the opposite side. Instruct the patient to grip both crutches by the handgrips. Help the patient to reach back with the free hand to find the arm of the chair. Instruct the patient to stretch the non-weight-bearing foot forward. Assist the patient with slowly lowering their weight into the chair.

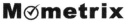

AMBULATING PATIENT WITH A WALKER

A patient who is learning to ambulate with a **walker** should wear a gait belt at all times. Instruct the patient to stand in the middle of the walker, holding it by the handgrips. Instruct the patient to move the walker forward until the back legs are even with the toes. While keeping their weight on the strong leg, the patient should then take a step forward with the weaker leg, until it is in the center of the walker. Then, instruct the patient to place their weight upon the handgrips while taking a step forward with the strong leg. Once the patient has regained balance, repeat the process.

ASSISTING PATIENT FROM SITTING POSITION TO STANDING WITH WALKER

While the patient is sitting in the chair, open the walker and place it in front of the patient. Make sure the patient is wearing a gait belt. Instruct the patient to scoot forward until they are sitting on the edge of the chair. Instruct the patient to place both hands on the arms of the chair. On the count of three, assist the patient into a standing position. While providing support for the patient, instruct them to move their hands, one at a time, from the arms of the chair to the handgrips of the walker. Wait a moment to ensure the patient is not dizzy before beginning to ambulate.

AMBULATING A PATIENT WITH A CANE

While ambulating a patient who is learning how to walk with a **cane**, always provide the patient with a gait belt. Instruct the patient to hold the cane in their strong hand. As the patient takes a step forward with the affected extremity, advance the cane forward, keeping the cane even with the leg and the patient's full weight upon their strong leg. Once the weakened leg and the cane are in place, instruct the patient to place their weight upon the cane while taking a step forward with the unaffected extremity. Allow the patient a moment to regain balance before repeating the process.

PATIENT POSITIONS

Specific patient positions are utilized for various procedures and conditions:

- When the patient is in a **supine** position, they are lying flat on the back, with arms extended at the sides.
- A **prone** position consists of the patient resting on the stomach, with the head turned to one side on the pillow and arms extended at the side.
- When the patient is in the **lateral** position, they should be positioned on their side, with both legs straight.
- **Sims'** position is similar to the lateral position in that the patient is lying on the side. However, in the Sims' position, the patient's topmost leg is flexed. Both the flexed leg and topmost arm are elevated on a pillow for additional support.
- The **semi-Fowler's** position consists of the patient lying on the back with the head of the bed at a 45° angle.
- A **high-Fowler's** position is similar to the semi-Fowler's, but the head of the bed is raised to a 90° angle.

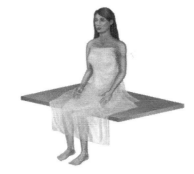

SEATED POSITION

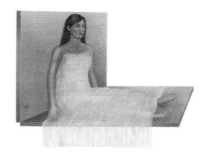

HIGH FOWLER'S POSITION

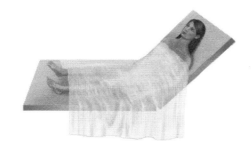

SEMI FOWLER'S POSITION

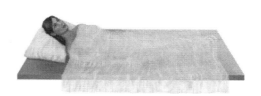

SUPINE POSITION

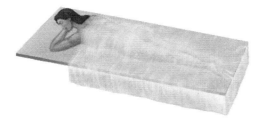

PRONE POSITION

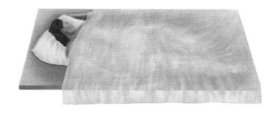

SIMS POSITION

MOVING THE PATIENT UP IN BED

Never try to move a patient up in bed by oneself. Always ask another nurse aide or nurse to help. Prior to moving the patient up in bed, explain to the patient what is going to be done. Wash hands and don a pair of gloves. Lay the head of the bed as flat as possible and raise the level of the bed until it is a comfortable height. Position oneself near the head of the bed on one side, while the other person moves to the opposite side of the bed. Instruct the patient to cross the arms over their chest to prevent limbs from dragging and to tuck the chin to the chest. If the patient is unable to do so, support the back of the neck with one hand. Grasp the draw sheet and roll the edge to establish a good grip. On the count of three, lift the draw sheet and pull upward. Position the patient for comfort.

PLACING A PATIENT INTO SIDE-LYING POSITION

Prior to turning a patient into a **side-lying position**, obtain assistance from a nurse or nurse aide. Raise the level of the bed to a comfortable height. Using the draw sheet, move the patient closer to the side of the bed opposite of the direction they will be turned; this will allow the patient to remain in the center of the bed after having been turned. Grasp the draw sheet and use it to pull the patient

35

onto their side. If the patient is able, ask them to grasp the side rail while they are being positioned. Tuck a pillow beneath the patient's back, under the draw sheet. Tuck another pillow beneath the patient's buttocks. Place a pillow underneath the patient's arm and between the patient's knees for support. Remove gloves and wash the hands.

LOGROLLING A PATIENT

Logrolling is a procedure that is performed whenever the patient has sustained a neck or spinal cord injury. Ideally, patients with this type of injury should be turned as little as possible until the neck or spine has been stabilized. In certain cases, turning cannot be avoided, such as if the patient has become incontinent. If the patient must be moved, the head, neck, and back must be kept in a stable position to prevent further injury. This requires good communication among the caregivers who are moving the patient to ensure that their movements are coordinated to maintain proper alignment.

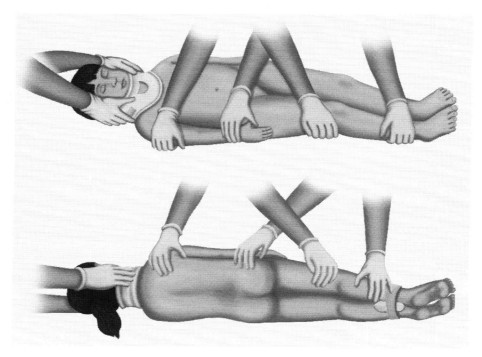

Logrolling a patient requires a minimum of three people in order to be performed successfully. The procedure is as follows:

1. Wash hands, don a pair of gloves, and explain what is going to be done.
2. Have one person positioned at the patient's head and two others on the side in which the patient is to be facing.
3. Grasp the draw sheet and turn the patient. The person at the head of the bed should keep the patient's head midline with the rest of the body, while the people at the side of the bed keep the back and hips in alignment.
4. Perform the necessary procedures and then return the patient to their back. It is imperative that the patient's head, neck, and back are kept in alignment.
5. Position the patient for comfort and wash hands.

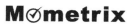

PERFORMING RANGE OF MOTION EXERCISES ON PATIENTS

IMPORTANCE OF PERFORMING RANGE OF MOTION ON PATIENTS

Patients who are bed bound are at an increased risk of muscle deterioration from lack of use. Lack of regular exercise also places patients at risk for developing contractures, a painful condition that results in the permanent shortening of the muscle or tendon. **Range-of-motion exercises** can be performed to maintain muscle tone during periods in which the patient lacks the strength to perform other forms of activity. Patients may also be assisted with performing range-of-motion activities if they are unable to do so themselves, such as in cases in which patients are sedated or comatose.

MOVEMENTS USED DURING RANGE OF MOTION EXERCISES

Specific **movements** used during ROM exercises can be described using the following terms:

- **Flexion** refers to bending at a joint, resulting in a decrease in the angle of the joint. For example, when the arm is bent at the elbow, it is flexed.
- **Extension** refers to the straightening of a joint, or increasing the angle of that joint. For example, when the arm is straightened, it is extended.
- **Abduction** refers to the movement away from the trunk. For example, when the arm is moved away from the body, such as during jumping jacks, it is abducted.
- **Adduction** refers to a movement that brings a limb closer to the trunk. For example, when the arm moves back toward the body, it is adducted.
- **Rotation** occurs when a part of the body pivots on a central axis. For example, when the head turns from side to side, it is considered to be rotating.

HOW TO PERFORM RANGE OF MOTION ON PATIENTS

Range-of-motion exercises are typically performed during the patient's bath. They can also be performed while the patient is sitting in a chair or lying in bed. Each exercise should be performed 10 times to ensure it is effective. The procedure is as follows:

1. Wash hands and explain to the patient what is going to be done.
2. Raise the level of the bed until it is a comfortable height.
3. Begin by performing range-of-motion exercises on the patient's head; instruct the patient to rotate the head from one side to the other. This exercise should not be performed on patients who have suffered neck or spinal cord injuries.
4. Work on the arms next. Flex and extend both arms at the elbow then abduct and adduct the arm. Flex and extend both wrists and all fingers.
5. Range of motion of the legs includes flexion and extension of the leg at the knee, as well as abduction and adduction of the leg.
6. Finally, flex and extend the ankles and toes.

37

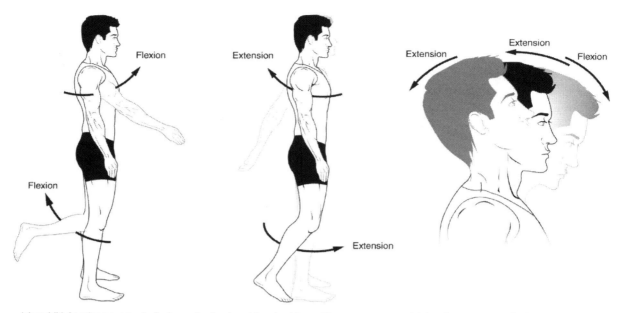

(a) and (b) Angular movements: flexion and extension at the shoulder and knees

(c) Angular movements: flexion and extension of the neck

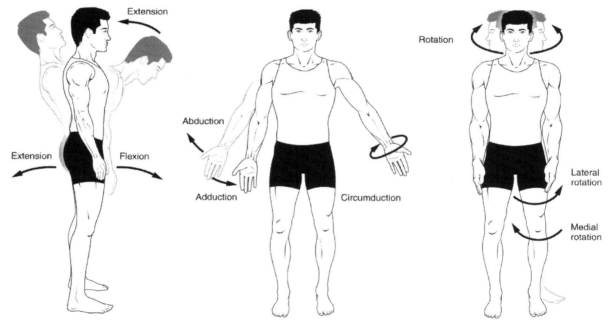

(d) Angular movements: flexion and extension of the vertebral column

(e) Angular movements: abduction, adduction, and circumduction of the upper limb at the shoulder

(f) Rotation of the head, neck, and lower limb

ACTIVE RANGE OF MOTION AND PASSIVE RANGE OF MOTION

Active range of motion (AROM) occurs when patients are able to perform range-of-motion activities by themselves. Though they may receive directions from the nurse aide, the patient performs the bulk of the exercise.

Passive range of motion (PROM) consists of the same exercises that are performed during AROM. PROM occurs when the nurse aide is performing range-of-motion activities on a sedated or

38

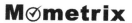

comatose patient to prevent muscle weakness. PROM may also be performed on patients whose muscle weakness is so pronounced that they require assistance in order to perform the activity.

ABNORMAL FINDINGS

Range-of-motion exercises should be performed at least once or twice every day to make sure the patient's joints do not become **contracted**. Stiffness or the inability to move the joint may be an indication of the onset of contractures; if either of these symptoms is noticed, they should be reported to the nurse immediately. While performing range of motion, the nursing aide should monitor for any signs of **swelling or inflammation** in the joints. If the patient experiences **sudden severe pain** or **respiratory distress** while performing range of motion, the nurse should be notified immediately.

BODY MECHANICS

PROPER BODY MECHANICS

Proper body mechanics are described as the safe completion of tasks using the appropriate muscle groups in order to avoid straining or injury. Health care workers have the highest incidences of work-related muscle injuries as a result of frequent heavy lifting, and these injuries are often slow to heal. Proper body mechanics are important in the medical field because of the frequent need to lift, turn, and reposition patients. Good body mechanics ensure the avoidance of using back muscles while caring for the patient, resulting in decreased fatigue and reduced risk of injury for both the patient and the nurse aide.

PRINCIPLES OF BODY MECHANICS

There are four **principles of body mechanics** that should be followed in order to avoid injury.

1. The first is to **maintain a proper center of gravity**. This is done by bending and lifting with the legs and keeping the back straight while lifting.
2. The second principle of body mechanics is to **maintain a wide base of support**, in order to maintain stability while lifting. Establish this wide base of support by keeping the feet at least 12 inches apart, with one foot slightly ahead of the other.
3. The third principle is to **maintain proper alignment**. While lifting a heavy object, keep the back straight and the item that is being lifted close to the body. If the nurse aide needs to turn with the object, the whole body should be pivoted rather than twisting with the object.
4. The fourth principle of body mechanics is to **maintain proper posture while lifting**. Keep the head up, the back straight, the knees flexed, and the buttocks tucked in to prevent injury while lifting.

DEEP VEIN THROMBOSIS (DVT)

A deep vein thrombosis (DVT), is a blood clot that develops in the larger veins in an extremity. DVTs most commonly form in the legs, though the risk of developing a DVT in the arms does increase if the patient has an intravenous line. DVTs are most commonly caused by immobilization, though other factors such as obesity, infection, tobacco use, and advanced age can increase the patient's risk for developing a clot. The most common signs of a DVT include swelling and redness of the affected extremity. The patient may also complain of pain in the affected extremity. DVTs present a heavy risk for embolism, when part of the clot breaks apart and travels in the bloodstream to the heart, lungs, or brain. This can result in pulmonary embolism, heart attack, or stroke. If a patient presents with any signs of a DVT, that extremity should be elevated and rubbing/massaging of the extremity should be avoided (as this can create an embolism). The nurse should be notified immediately.

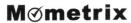

SEQUENTIAL COMPRESSION DEVICE (SCD)

A sequential compression device (SCD) is a pair of cuffs that are placed on the patient's legs to prevent the formation of blood clots. While the SCDs are on, the device applies pressure to different parts of the legs over time. The increased pressure encourages blood flow within the legs, preventing blood clots. Care should be taken while the SCDs are in place to ensure the tubing does not become kinked as this prevents the SCDs from working. The circulation in the patient's feet should also be monitored. Frequent skin care should be performed as the skin underneath the cuffs can become damp and hot. SCDs should not be used on extremities that have an existing DVT, as it could encourage the formation of an embolism.

ANTI-EMBOLISM STOCKINGS AND ELASTIC BANDAGES

ANTI-EMBOLISM STOCKINGS

Anti-embolism stockings or T.E.D. (thrombo-embolic deterrent) hose are tight elastic stockings that are applied to the patient's legs. They are typically prescribed for patients who have undergone surgery or have decreased activity. When a patient is unable to move, blood pools in the legs, which increases the risk of developing blood clots and edema. Anti-embolism stockings work by placing pressure on the legs, which encourages blood flow. With improved circulation in the lower extremities, the patient's risk for developing a blood clot or edema is decreased. Care should be taken to frequently monitor circulation in the patient's legs while the anti-embolism stockings are in place.

APPLYING ANTI-EMBOLISM STOCKINGS

The process for applying anti-embolism stockings is as follows:

1. Prior to applying anti-embolism stockings, verify that the anti-embolism stockings are the proper size for the patient based upon height and weight; they should be tight without cutting off circulation.
2. Place the patient in a supine position.
3. Gather the fabric of the anti-embolism stocking and slide it onto the patient's foot.
4. Roll the stocking upward until the upper edge is placed above the patient's knee.
5. Check to make sure there are no wrinkles in the stocking and that the stocking is placed properly so that the toes and heels are in the appropriate spots.
6. Once the stocking is in place, position the patient for comfort, remove the gloves, and wash hands.

APPLYING ELASTIC BANDAGES

The process for applying elastic bandages is as follows:

1. Prior to applying an elastic bandage, check the order to confirm where the bandage is to be placed.
2. Wash the hands and apply a pair of gloves.
3. Hold the end of the bandage in place with one hand and wrap it around the extremity twice to secure it.
4. Continue to wrap the bandage around the area that needs to be covered, working from bottom to top.
5. While wrapping, overlap the bandages to keep them from sliding down and to ensure the area is covered.
6. Once the elastic bandage is in place, secure it with tape, clips, or Velcro.
7. Remove the gloves and wash hands.

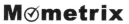

Monitoring Patients Wearing Elastic Bandages or Anti-Embolism Stockings

While patients are wearing anti-embolism stockings or elastic bandages, it is important to **monitor** them closely to ensure they receive an appropriate amount of circulation to their extremities. Frequently assess the patient's toes (or fingers, if the elastic bandage is on the arm) to check for signs of decreased circulation. Any complaints of numbness, tingling, or decreased sensation in the extremity should be reported to the nurse and investigated immediately. Make sure to remove the patient's anti-embolism stockings every 8 hours to allow for circulation. Elastic bandages should be removed per the doctor's order.

Pressure Ulcers

Stages

Pressure ulcers are divided into **stages**, classified by the depth of the wound.

Stage	Description
Stage I	An area of redness that is typically located over a bony prominence. The reddened area may feel painful or warm to the touch.
Stage II	The wearing away of the first layer of skin, revealing a pink wound bed below.
Stage III	An ulcer that extends past the full thickness of the skin into the subcutaneous tissue; fatty tissue may be visualized. Tunneling may also be present.
Stage IV	A loss of enough skin tissue to reveal muscle tissue or bone.
Unstageable	The wound bed is covered with necrotic (dead, black) tissue and therefore cannot be visualized/assessed to stage.

Prevention

There are a number of methods available to **prevent** the formation of pressure ulcers.

- The primary method of prevention is **frequent repositioning**. The patient should be turned and repositioned at least every two hours to prevent skin breakdown. Pillows may be used to provide additional support.
- The patient's **feet should be elevated** to prevent breakdown on the ankles, and the head of the bed should be kept at less than a 30° angle to reduce pressure on the buttocks.
- The patient's **skin should be assessed** frequently.
- The patient's **nutritional status** should be closely monitored as well since patients who have poor nutrition are at an increased risk of developing a pressure sore.

Air Mattresses and Egg Crate Mattresses

Pressure ulcers typically develop when the patient is unable to move as a result of illness or injury. As the patient lies in bed, their weight causes breakdown over bony prominences, such as over the shoulder blades and coccyx. When inflated, an **air mattress** decreases the amount of pressure placed upon the bony prominences. An **egg crate mattress** is a foam cushion that has alternating raised areas and grooves that decrease the area of pressure on bony prominences. Though these items do not replace turning the patient, they can aid in preventing pressure sores in high-risk patients.

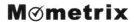

TREATMENT

Pressure ulcers are difficult to heal as a result of the patient's compromised health status. If a patient develops a pressure ulcer, it is important to ensure it does not get worse by frequently turning and repositioning the patient. The patient should be placed on a support surface, such as an air mattress. This helps to decrease the amount of pressure on bony prominences. The skin over the affected area should be kept clean and dry. Dressings can be applied to the pressure sore, though the type of dressing depends on the severity of the pressure ulcer. It is also important to ensure the patient maintains good nutrition to ensure healing.

CARING FOR A PATIENT WITH CONTRACTURES

Patients that are immobile have a high risk for **contractures**, the permanent shortening of muscles/tendons that results in frozen joints and deformities. There are a number of treatment options for a patient with contractures. When a patient first develops a contracture, the nurse and the physical therapist should be notified. Attempts should be made to mobilize the joint using range-of-motion techniques. Heat therapy may be used prior to initiating activity to ease pain and increase flexibility. In some cases, the affected joint may be placed in a splint, which will continuously stretch the joint. Care of the splint should be performed as ordered by the doctor. If the contracture does not respond to other treatments, the patient may be taken to surgery to manipulate the tendon.

PREVENTING EDEMA

Edema can develop in the patient's extremities as a result of fluid overload or inactivity. The nurse aide can prevent swelling by encouraging the patient to move. If the patient is unable to walk, range-of-motion exercises should be frequently performed. While in bed or in the chair, the patient's legs should be elevated on pillows to prevent swelling in the lower extremities. Massaging the patient's extremities using lotion can also prevent edema. If the patient has a history of heart or kidney failure, their fluid and sodium intake should be closely monitored, as too much can result in increased edema.

EFFECTS OF IMMOBILITY ON SELF-IMAGE AND ACTIVITY TOLERANCE

Patients may be immobile for a number of reasons, including edema, weakness, trauma, pain, severe infection, and neuromuscular disease. **Immobility** prevents the patient from interacting normally with the environment and others, so the patient may become focused on body and health concerns, becoming demanding or, in some cases, passive. The patient may begin to feel powerless because of the necessity of relying on others to meet needs and may develop a negative body image and lowered self-esteem. The patient may become depressed, angry, and withdrawn, especially if immobility is prolonged.

Additionally, immobility interferes with the patient's ability to carry out activities of daily living without assistance. Muscles weaken from disuse, bones lose calcium and are more prone to fractures, and the patient may experience a sudden fall in blood pressure when sitting or standing (orthostatic hypotension). The patient may tire easily and is at increased risk of falls.

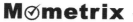

Basic Nursing Skills

CARING FOR VISUALLY IMPAIRED PATIENTS

A nurse aide should take special precautions when caring for a patient who has a **visual impairment**. Prior to interacting with the patient, the nurse aide should become acquainted with the type of visual impairment the patient has. Aides should make sure to identify themselves as soon as they enter the room and stand within the patient's visual field while interacting with him or her. While ambulating the patient, the nurse aide should allow the patient to move as freely as possible and provide clear verbal cues regarding potential obstacles. The furniture in the patient's room should not be moved to allow the patient to become familiar with the surroundings.

CARING FOR HEARING IMPAIRED PATIENTS

If the patient has **difficulty hearing** in one ear, the nurse aide should talk while standing on the side that the patient can hear from. The nurse aide should introduce oneself and speak slowly and clearly. The nurse aide should face the patient while talking to give the opportunity to read lips. While talking to the patient, the nurse aide should try to limit background noise and deepen the tone of the voice in order to make the aide better heard. If the patient can see well, communication can be achieved using written messages rather than speaking.

CARING FOR PATIENTS WITH APHASIA

Aphasia is defined as difficulty speaking that results from lesions on the brain. Aphasia is typically caused by cerebral vascular accident, brain injury, brain tumors, or by progressive diseases, such as Alzheimer's disease or Parkinson's disease. Aphasia can come in a number of different forms. The patient may be unable to speak or may speak using inappropriate words and phrases. The patient may become unable to name objects or call objects by the wrong names. Aphasia can also affect the patient's ability to comprehend language. With aphasia, the patient may become unable to read, write, or form complete sentences.

Prior to interacting with the patient, the nurse aide should become acquainted with the type of aphasia the patient has and communicate with the patient accordingly. The key to caring for a patient with aphasia is to avoid becoming frustrated. Do not rush the patient; allow them time to gather their thoughts and say what they are trying to say. Avoid attempting to speak for the patient. Try to use a picture or letter board to assist with communication. If possible, allow the patient to write messages in order to communicate.

CARING FOR PATIENTS WITH CHANGES IN MOBILITY OR PARALYSIS

Patients with a **change in mobility** or **paralysis** may need a number of interventions to ensure safety and wellbeing, including the following:

- The patient's position should be changed at least every 2 hours with the limbs and back supported with pillows if in bed.
- The patient's skin should be examined every time patient is turned and when bathing to note any reddened or pressure areas.
- The patient should be taught to change positions and reminded if able to do so independently.
- Lotions or creams should be applied to skin to keep skin supple.
- Assistive devices should be used to move or transfer the patient and to assist with ambulation when necessary.

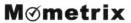

- The call light should be positioned where the patient is able to access it or an alternative method of alerting nurses should be provided.
- Assistance during meals may include providing assistive devices or feeding patient, depending on the degree of disability.
- Clothing/shoes be modified so that the patient can dress independently (Velcro openings, elastic shoe laces).
- Pressure-reducing devices may be needed in beds and chairs.
- Range of motion exercises should be done daily.

CARING FOR A PATIENT WEARING A CAST

Patients who are wearing a **cast** must be monitored closely to ensure they have continued circulation. Reasons for concern should be immediately reported to the nurse and include the following:

- If the fingers or toes of the extremity with the cast become cool, pale, or bluish in color, decreased perfusion due to a tight cast or swelling may be indicated.
- Sudden severe pain, numbness, or tingling may be an indication of poor circulation or nerve damage.
- A foul smell or a burning sensation coming from beneath the cast may be an indication of infection.

CONTRIBUTING TO PAIN MANAGEMENT

The nurse aide's responsibility in contributing to **pain management** begins with knowledge of both verbal and nonverbal expressions of pain and discomfort and prompt reporting of these observations to the appropriate licensed nurse (LVN/LPN or RN) so that a prescribed analgesia can be provided if necessary. The nurse aid can also help to relieve a patient's discomfort through comfort measures, which can include the following:

- Asking the patient what comfort measures will help to relieve the discomfort if the patient is alert and responsive
- Repositioning the patient and supporting the patient's body and limbs in good alignment with pillows/bolsters
- Providing a warm blanket
- Talking to the patient, showing concern, empathy, and support
- Providing aids to relaxation (music, white noise)
- Providing distraction: TV, music, reading, and activities (playing cards, working puzzles)
- Gently massaging the patient's back
- Providing a relaxing environment (lowering the lights, reducing noise)
- Assisting the patient with relaxation and visualization exercises

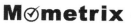

Infection Control

LOCALIZED VS. SYSTEMIC INFECTION

Infections are divided into two groups, localized and systemic.

- A **localized infection** occurs when a virus or bacteria begins to grow in a small area of the body. This can occur in wounds or surgical sites if not treated properly. Signs and symptoms of a localized infection include warmth, redness, and swelling around the site; purulent or foul-smelling drainage; or a fever.
- In a **systemic infection**, a virus or bacteria has gained access to the bloodstream, spreading to other parts of the body as a result. Signs of a systemic infection include fever, malaise, nausea, vomiting, chills, and generalized weakness. Systemic infection can lead to sepsis and, if not treated promptly, death.

BACTERIAL VS. VIRAL INFECTION

A **bacterial infection** is caused when bacteria are introduced into the body. The bacteria multiply to infect the patient, resulting in infection. Bacterial infection is typically localized. For example, a throat infection may result in worse pain on one side of the throat. Antibiotics must be prescribed to help kill bacterial growth as these infections do not tend to resolve on their own.

Viral infections occur when a virus invades the body through the mucous membranes. It attaches itself to a living cell and uses its genetic material to produce more of the virus. This results in the death of the host cell. Viral infections do not respond to antibiotic treatment. Though some antiviral medications exist, the usual course of treatment in a viral infection is to treat the symptoms and bolster the immune system to fight the infection. Some serious viral infections are controlled through the use of vaccinations to bolster the body's immune system against a specific virus, providing the body with the appropriate defenses to recognize and kill the virus upon entry. The FDA has approved vaccinations for influenza, measles, mumps, rubella, and polio, amongst others.

TRANSMISSION OF MICROORGANISMS

Microorganisms must move from one host to another in order to survive. There are various means of **transmission of microorganisms**:

- Some microorganisms are transmitted via **droplets** or **aerosols** that are released when an infected host coughs or sneezes. The microorganisms in the droplets/aerosols can then invade a new host via the mucous membranes of the eyes, nose, or mouth.
- Microorganisms may also be transmitted through **direct oral contact**, such as through kissing an infected person or by drinking from the same cup as the sick individual.
- **Iatrogenic transmission** occurs when microorganisms move to a new host during a medical procedure, such as a surgery or line placement.
- On rare occasions, microorganisms can be transmitted through the **fecal-oral route**. This most typically occurs as a result of indirect contact with fecal material, such as through poor hand washing or by eating foods that have been contaminated.

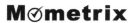

UNIVERSAL PRECAUTIONS

Universal precautions involve treating all patient secretions as if they contain a pathogen, resulting in the avoidance of direct contact with any secretions. **Universal precautions** are practiced in the health care setting whenever there is the risk of coming into contact with blood or body fluids. The precautions include wearing gloves when collecting blood or handling anything that may have been contaminated with blood. Use of other protective equipment may be necessary, such as wearing a face shield when suctioning copious secretions or a facemask to protect oneself from airborne secretions. If blood or body fluids have contaminated a work surface, it should be cleaned using the appropriate disinfectant.

HAND WASHING
PURPOSE

Microorganisms are present on all surfaces and can be transferred via touch. Certain microorganisms can cause illness or infection if they come into contact with a person whose immune system has been compromised. As a result, **hand washing** is a vital part of infection control. If properly done, hand washing removes visible dirt and germs from the hands. It prevents transmission of germs from the nurse aide to the patient or from one patient to another patient. Warm water, antimicrobial soap, and firm friction applied to all areas of the hand while washing are key factors in ensuring that the hands are clean and free of germs.

PROPER PROCEDURE

The proper procedure for washing the hands with soap and water is as follows:

1. Before beginning to wash, remove any jewelry on the hands and wrists.
2. Run the water until it is warm and then wet the hands to the wrist.
3. Apply a small amount of soap. Continue to work the soap into a lather for at least 30 seconds, using firm friction between the fingers, underneath the fingernails, and up the wrists.
4. Make sure to keep the hands lower than the elbows to prevent germs from traveling up the arm.
5. If the hands have been soiled with body fluids, hand washing should be performed for at least one minute.
6. Rinse hands thoroughly with warm water and then dry the hands.
7. When the hands are dry, use part of the towel to turn the faucet off.

Proper hand washing is the key to infection control. Because germs run off the hands while hand washing is performed, it is important to ensure that hands do not touch the inside of the sink while washing. If a nurse aide's hands touch the inside of the sink, then hand washing should be repeated to ensure the hands have not become contaminated. The wet surface of bar soap can provide a medium for germs to grow. Prior to beginning to wash hands, rub the soap vigorously to remove the outermost layer of soap. Then, once hand washing has been completed, rinse the soap with warm water.

ALCOHOL-BASED HAND SANITIZER

Alcohol-based hand sanitizers have been approved as an adjunct to hand washing in the health care setting. They work by removing the outer layer of oils on the hand, killing any bacteria on the hand in the process. To use hand sanitizer, take a dime-sized amount into the dominant hand. Rub the hands together vigorously for at least thirty seconds. Make sure to rub between the fingers, between the knuckles, and beneath the fingernails. If, after thirty seconds, the hands are still damp, allow them to air dry. Once the hands have dried, they are considered clean.

46

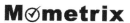

WASHING HANDS INSTEAD OF USING ALCOHOL SCRUB

There are instances in which hand washing is indicated over use of an alcohol-based hand sanitizer:

- Even if hand sanitizer is used appropriately, hands should occasionally be washed to remove any residue that can build up as a result of frequent use of alcohol scrub.
- The nurse aide should wash their hands with soap and water if they have been soiled with secretions (blood, urine, saliva/sputum, vomit, feces, oral secretions, etc.).
- Hand washing should be used prior to eating and after using the bathroom.
- Hand washing is required after caring for patients infected with *clostridium difficile*, an infectious bacterium that is not effectively killed with alcohol-based hand sanitizer.

PPE

Types of personal protective equipment (PPE) include the following:

- **Gloves** are the most commonly used piece of protective equipment in the health care setting. They are typically made of thin vinyl or nitrile rubber and are intended for single use. They should be used whenever there is a risk of touching infectious material or body fluids.
- **Gowns** are typically made of thin plastic or synthetic waterproof fibers. They are typically worn over the uniform whenever the patient is in contact isolation or when splashes by bodily fluids is possible.
- **Face protection** options include the following:
  - **Facemasks** are worn over the nose and mouth to prevent inhalation of infectious material.
  - **Goggles** are worn over the eyes to prevent introduction of infectious materials to the eyes.
  - When dealing with a large amount of secretions, a **face shield** can be worn in place of a facemask and goggles.

DONNING AND DOFFING PPE

Isolation equipment should be **donned** before entering an isolation room. The order of donning PPE is as follows:

1. The **gown** should be unfolded and held with the opening toward the back. Place the arms through the sleeves. Tie the gown securely behind the neck and at the waist.
2. Next, the **facemask** should be applied making sure both the nose and mouth are covered.
3. Finally, **gloves** should be applied and worn so they cover the cuffs of the isolation gown.

Isolation gear should be **removed (doffed)** prior to leaving the room in the following order:

1. The **gloves** should be removed first. Grasp the first glove at the wrist and pull to remove it. Then ball the used glove in the hand that is still gloved. Grasp the remaining glove at the wrist and pull to remove it.
2. Next, remove the **gown** and the **mask**.
3. Once the gloves, gown, and mask have been removed, **wash hands**.

BASIC PRECAUTIONS FOR CHANGING LINENS

When changing linens, the nurse aide should wear gloves and avoid holding the linens close to the body. Soiled linens should not be shaken out, as this may release germs into the air. Once all of the soiled linens have been removed from the bed and put into the appropriate receptacle, the nurse aide should remove his or her gloves and wash hands. The aide should then securely tie the linen bag closed and place it in the soiled utility room. Clean linens should be carefully unfolded and placed on the bed. Any linen that has fallen on the floor should be considered contaminated; it should be placed in the soiled utility bin and replaced with clean linen.

ISOLATION

Isolation refers to special measures taken to prevent the spread of germs. The goal is to protect other patients and hospital staff while providing care to the patient. Isolation may be required if the patient has a particularly infectious disease, such as tuberculosis or Varicella. The patient may also be placed into isolation if they have a drug-resistant bacterium, such as methicillin-resistant *staphylococcus aureus* (MRSA) or *clostridium difficile* (*C. diff*). Depending upon the type of isolation, the nurse aide may be required to wear an isolation gown, gloves, and/or a mask while providing care for the patient.

ISOLATION PRECAUTIONS

There are three types of isolation precautions:

- **Contact precautions** are intended to limit the spread of microorganisms that might be transmitted by direct contact with a contaminated surface. If a patient is in contact isolation, they should be in a private room that is clearly marked. When providing care to the patient, the nurse aide should wear an isolation gown and gloves at all times while in the room.
- **Droplet precautions** are intended to limit the spread of microorganisms that are transmitted via mucous or respiratory secretions. A patient who requires droplet precautions should be placed in a private room. A nurse aide should wear a mask and gloves when caring for a patient who is in droplet precautions.
- **Airborne precautions** are intended to prevent the spread of airborne microorganisms that can survive for long periods of time in the environment. While on airborne precautions, the patient should be placed in a negative pressure room. While caring for the patient, the nurse aide should wear an appropriately fitting N95 mask or respirator and gloves.

REQUIRED ITEMS FOR ISOLATION PATIENTS

The nurse aide should take care to ensure that germs from a patient in isolation are not spread amid the patient population. A cart should be placed outside of the patient's room containing isolation equipment that should be donned prior to entering the room. This includes waterproof isolation gowns, gloves, and masks, as well as a garbage bag for waste disposal. Germicidal wipes should also be available to clean the equipment that must be shared with the rest of the patient population. The patient in isolation can also be provided with disposable equipment that might ordinarily be shared among the patient population, such as single-use stethoscopes and blood pressure cuffs.

SPECIAL REMOVAL OF SOILED LINEN FROM AN ISOLATION ROOM

Care must be taken while **removing soiled linen** from an isolation room. Because the linen bag was in the isolation room, it is considered contaminated. The soiled linen bag must be placed inside a clean bag to prevent contamination. While the nurse aide is bathing the patient, soiled linen should be placed in a plastic linen bag. Once bathing has been completed, the linen bag should be tied securely shut. Another aide standing outside the door should hold a second linen bag open while the first bag is placed inside; the second bag should also be tied securely shut. The double-bagged linen bag should be left outside while the nurse aide removes their isolation gown, gloves, and mask, and washes the hands. Then, the soiled linen can be taken to the soiled utility room.

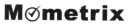

EQUIPMENT MAINTENANCE
INFECTION FROM PATIENT CARE EQUIPMENT

The level of risk for infection from patient care equipment refers to the likelihood that a piece of equipment will contain infectious pathogens on its surface; it aids in determining the proper level of cleaning prior to subsequent use.

- **Low-risk or noncritical items** are pieces of equipment that come into contact with intact skin, such as stethoscopes. Noncritical items also include inanimate objects in the environment, such as countertops and walls. These items only require cleaning with a detergent prior to subsequent use.
- **Intermediate-risk or semi-critical items** are those that come in close contact with mucous membranes but do not penetrate the skin, such as thermometers or respiratory equipment. These items require cleaning with a high-level disinfectant before they are ready for use.
- **High-risk or critical items**, such as surgical instruments and devices, have penetrated or will penetrate the skin and are at high risk for contamination by microorganisms. These items require sterilization before they are ready for subsequent use.

CLEANING, DISINFECTION, AND STERILIZATION

Cleaning refers to the process that removes visible dirt or soiled material from a surface. It typically involves using water or a detergent to rinse the surface. Cleaning must be performed prior to disinfection or sterilization.

Disinfection is defined as the process that destroys most microorganisms on the surface of a piece of equipment. The disinfectant that is used is typically chemical in nature, though some pieces of equipment may be disinfected using heat.

Sterilization refers to the process that removes all forms of microbial life from a piece of equipment.

PROCESS FOR CLEANING EQUIPMENT

Cleaning refers to the process of removing dirt or organic material from the surface of a piece of equipment. If an item is not properly cleaned, subsequent disinfection or sterilization may not be effective. Gloves should be worn while cleaning equipment. Thoroughly wipe each piece of equipment with a detergent, rubbing with firm pressure to remove any dirt or organic material. Once the organic material and dirt has been removed, rinse the surface thoroughly with water and allow it to dry prior to subsequent use. Hand washing should be performed after cleaning any equipment.

PROCESS FOR STERILIZING EQUIPMENT

Sterilization requires a piece of equipment be exposed to extreme dry heat or a chemical sterilant to remove all microorganisms. Equipment is typically exposed to dry heat during the autoclaving process. Autoclaving is considered to be the most effective method of sterilization. Chemical sterilization is used for equipment unable to tolerate high temperatures, such as fluids and rubber. Care must be taken when handling sterile equipment. Any contact with a non-sterile surface will introduce new microorganisms to the equipment. When a piece of sterile equipment is prepared for use, it should be handled using sterile technique.

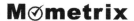

Patient Safety

PATIENT FALLS
RISK FACTORS AND PREVENTION

Patient falls are a considerable problem in the health care setting. Injuries resulting from a fall are considered to be a primary cause of morbidity in older adults. The loss of coordination and bone density as people age puts them at an increased risk for breaking bones after a fall; the resultant loss of independence may lead to a decline in health and eventual death. Yet falling is not a normal part of aging. Proper **prevention** can greatly decrease a patient's risk of falling. As a nurse aide, it is important to follow fall precautions to prevent patient falls within the hospital setting.

NECESSARY PRECAUTIONS

There are a number of **precautions** that can be taken to prevent patient falls. The first step of prevention is identifying the needs of the patient. If the patient has been determined to be a fall risk, a sign should be placed on the door so the staff knows the patient has special mobility needs. While the patient is in bed, at least two side rails should be kept in the raised position to prevent the patient from falling out of bed. Prior to standing with assistance, patients should be allowed to sit or dangle at the side of the bed to prevent dizziness that may result from the change in position. The patient should also wear rubber-soled shoes or socks. The floor should be kept free of all hazards, including puddles of water and small rugs that can cause slipping. While the patient sits in or stands up from the chair or wheelchair, the brakes should be kept locked.

SAFETY PRECAUTIONS FOR BED-BOUND PATIENTS

Patients who are **bedridden** have a particularly high risk of falling. While the patient is in bed, make sure the side rails are up to prevent the patient from climbing out of bed. If necessary, a bed alarm may be placed in the bed to alert the nurse aide that the patient is attempting to get out of bed without assistance. The patient's call light should be placed within reach, as well as the patient's tray table and any other items the patient might need. Toileting should be offered at least every two hours, and the patient should be turned every two hours to prevent bedsores.

PROPER TECHNIQUE FOR FALLING WITH A PATIENT

Even with all necessary precautions properly observed while ambulating, the patient is still at risk for falling. A fall may result if the patient's legs give out from under them or if they were to lose consciousness while ambulating. If a sudden fall were to occur, it is important to protect the patient and oneself from harm. Support the patient using the gait belt and the free arm, and gently lower the patient to the floor or to a nearby chair, taking care to protect the patient's head. If the fall is uncontrolled as a result of loss of balance, focus on supporting the patient as much as possible while keeping oneself safe. Try to avoid tensing up prior to impact as this may cause additional injury.

COMMON DEVICES USED TO PROMOTE PATIENT SAFETY

Common devices used to promote patient safety include the following:

- **Lifts**: Utilizing lifts, such as the Hoyer lift, to assist in moving and lifting patients reduces the risk of falls and injuries.
- **Assistive devices**: Various assistive devices, such as canes, walkers, wheelchairs, grabbers, reaching devices, and medication dispensers, help to prevent falls, facilitate mobility, and promote safety.

Copyright © Mometrix Media. You have been licensed one copy of this document for personal use only. Any other reproduction or redistribution is strictly prohibited. All rights reserved. This content is provided for test preparation purposes only and does not imply an endorsement by Mometrix of any particular political, scientific, or religious point of view.

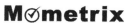

- **Alarms**: Many types of sensors with alarms are available, including floor mat sensors, chair sensors, seatbelt sensors, and movement sensors. Door alarms may sound when doors are opened to alert staff.
- **Wander management systems**: Systems such as *Wanderguard* and *RoamAlert* require the patient to wear a device (such as a bracelet) that contains a locator and may also have a door controller to automatically lock doors as the patient approaches them or to sound alarm if the patient passes through an open door.

RESTRAINTS
TYPES
There are a number of different types of **restraints** that can be used in a health care setting.

- **Emotional restraints** are a method of using verbal or emotional cues in order to attempt to modify the patient's behaviors. This can include limit setting or contracting with the patient for safety.
- **Environmental restraints** are devices used to restrict patient movement. These include side-rails on the bed or locked doors within the facility. When all four side-rails are in a raised position on the bed, it is considered to be a restraint.
- **Physical restraints** are devices that can be applied to the patient to restrict movement. These include wrist and vest restraints, lap belts, and movement pads.
- **Chemical restraints** are medications that are given to the patient to modify behavior.

PURPOSE
Restraint policies vary from one facility to another, but their **purpose** remains the same. Restraints are applied in order to protect the patient from causing harm to oneself or to other people. A restraint may be applied to prevent the patient from interfering with medical devices or moving in a way that would be detrimental to their health. It may also be applied if the patient is showing signs of aggression. A restraint should always be applied after all other alternatives have been exhausted. It should not be applied as a form of punishment or for the convenience of the staff.

CONSIDERATIONS PRIOR TO APPLYING RESTRAINTS
Prior to applying a restraint, all other alternatives must be exhausted. The health care staff must attempt to identify and address the behaviors that require the application of restraints. An order from the patient's physician must be obtained in order to apply restraints, and the physician should visibly assess the patient within 24 hours of the time of application of the restraints. Consent should be obtained from the patient's next of kin or power of attorney (POA). Care must be taken to choose the least restrictive form of restraint. The type of restraint should be explained to the patient, as well as the reasons for the application of the restraint and the requirements for removal of the restraint.

ALTERNATIVES TO RESTRAINTS
There are a number of measures that can be performed as an **alternative** to applying restraints. The type of alternatives that are utilized may vary depending upon the patient. Any needs should be assessed and all reasonable alternatives performed prior to application of restraints.

- The patient may need to be moved to a **quiet environment**.
- The patient may require **more stimulation**, such as hearing a television or radio in the background.
- The patient may require **redirection**.
- The patient may need **toileting or water**.

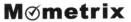

- The patient may need **personal items** placed within reach.
- The patient may require **distraction** if the care team is attempting to remove a medical device.
- If the patient has an **illness** or requires **rest**, it may cause them to act in a manner that is confused or inappropriate.

APPLYING RESTRAINTS TO EXTREMITIES

Extremity restraints are applied to the arms and legs to restrict movement. A doctor's order and consent from the family or POA must be obtained prior to application of these restraints. The nurse aide should wash their hands and don a pair of gloves. The nurse aide should then greet the patient and explain the need for the restraint, as well as the requirements for removal. The restraint should be applied per the manufacturer's instructions and tied to the frame of the bed using a quick release knot. The patient should be given a reasonable amount of slack in order to move. The nurse aide should be able to fit two fingers between the patient's extremity and the restraint; this ensures that is it not too tight.

VEST RESTRAINT

A vest restraint is a device that is placed over the patient's chest to restrict movement. It is typically applied to prevent a patient from getting up without assistance. A doctor's order and consent from the family/POA must be obtained prior to application of the restraint. The nurse aide should wash the hands and don a pair of gloves. The vest restraint should be placed on the patient so that the opening is toward the back, with the straps crossing in the back. The straps should then be tied with a quick release knot directly to the chair or the frame of the bed. At least two fingers should be able to fit beneath the vest restraint to ensure that it is not too tight. Once the restraint has been applied, remove the gloves and wash the hands. Monitor the patient per facility policy.

MONITORING PATIENT IN RESTRAINTS

Patients who are in restraints should be closely **monitored to ensure safety**. They should be checked frequently to make sure there is proper circulation. While they are restrained, patients should have their legs covered with a blanket in order to maintain privacy. The restraint should be removed every 2 hours to allow for range of motion. Patients should also be repositioned for comfort and offered water and toileting every two hours. Teaching regarding the restraints should be frequently reinforced to encourage patient understanding of the need for the restraint and the requirements for removal.

SECURING RESTRAINTS

When securing restraints on a patient who is in a wheelchair, care should be taken to ensure that the restraint is tied using a quick release knot attached directly to the frame of the wheelchair. The wheelchair should be locked, and care should be taken to ensure the restraints are not tied to the wheels. Similarly, when the patient is in bed, the restraint should be tied using a quick release knot attached directly to the frame of the bed. Tying the restraint to the side rail can cause injury to the patient if the side rail should fall.

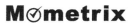

Emergencies

ENSURING FIRE SAFETY

Fire safety is very important in both the hospital and extended-care facility. Because of the presence of highly flammable materials, such as oxygen tanks, proper fire safety must be closely observed. The nurse aide should make note of the presence of oxygen shutoff valves, fire alarms, and fire extinguishers, and know the facility policy regarding fire alarms. Regular fire drills should be performed, and residents should be aware of necessary fire safety precautions. The fire extinguishers should be serviced regularly to ensure proper functioning. The nurse aide should also be aware of the facility code that indicates a fire. Though a fire is typically announced as a "Code Red" on the overhead speakers, individual facilities may have different alarm codes.

PASS

PASS is a mnemonic that refers to the proper way to handle a fire extinguisher:

Pull	A plastic ring keeps the fire extinguisher from being discharged accidentally. Pull the plastic ring off the fire extinguisher to make it ready for use.
Aim	Aim the nozzle of the fire extinguisher at the base of the fire.
Squeeze	Squeeze the trigger of the fire extinguisher to start the flow.
Sweep	Sweep the nozzle from side to side, covering the area of the fire completely. Continue to aim at the base of the fire, and do not stop the flow of fluid until the fire has been extinguished.

RACE

RACE is a mnemonic that explains the proper procedure that should be performed upon discovery of a fire within the hospital or extended-care facility:

Rescue	The first priority is to remove any patients who are in immediate danger from the fire. The nurse aide should only attempt to rescue a patient if it can be done without placing oneself in imminent danger.
Alert	Once any patients have been removed from danger, the nurse aide should activate the fire alarm system, if it has not already been done.
Contain	Fire doors should be closed in an attempt to deprive the fire of oxygen.
Extinguish	If it is safe to do so, attempt to extinguish the fire using the appropriate fire extinguisher.

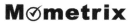

FIRE EXTINGUISHERS

There are multiple types of **fire extinguishers** that are typically found in a hospital or extended-care facility. The most common are the following:

- The first type is a **type A** fire extinguisher. It is typically silver in color and shoots pressurized water. Type A fire extinguishers are intended for ordinary combustibles, such as paper, wood, or cloth.
- A **type C** fire extinguisher shoots dry chemicals. It is typically red in color and is intended for fires started from an electrical source, such as a frayed wire or a piece of faulty equipment.
- The third type of fire extinguisher is the most commonly seen; it is referred to as a **type ABC** or multipurpose fire extinguisher. These are also red in color and are intended for fires that have been started by either a combustible, liquid chemical, or electrical source.

Before using a fire extinguisher, it is important to make note of which type of fire extinguisher is being used; a Type A fire extinguisher should not be used on an electrical fire.

EMERGENCY TREATMENT FOR BURNS

Depending on the severity and the amount of body surface it covers, a **burn** can be a life-threatening injury. Shock induced by a burn and the resulting impairment of the immune system can cause serious harm to the patient. It is important to act quickly if the patient has been severely burned. A burn that extends over a small area of the body should be treated by running cool water over the affected area. A sterile dressing should be applied over the burn to protect the skin and to prevent the introduction of germs. Ice packs should also be applied to protect the skin and nerve endings.

ENSURING ELECTRICAL SAFETY FOR FIRE PREVENTION

Proper **electrical safety** is an important step in fire prevention. The maintenance department should regularly service all patient care equipment. The nurse aide should regularly check to make sure that all equipment is within its maintenance period. If a piece of equipment appears to be malfunctioning, it should be removed from service immediately. Prior to a piece of equipment being used, it should be checked carefully to make sure its wires are intact. When plugging in a piece of equipment, make sure the circuits are not being overloaded. Also, closely monitor the floor near a piece of equipment to make sure there are no puddles nearby.

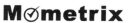

HOSPITAL EMERGENCY AND DISASTER RESPONSE PROTOCOL

Disaster/emergency response plans should be in place for the facility based on the Hospital Incident Command System (HICS), which provides a model for management, responsibilities, and communication. Disasters can include a multi-casualty influx of individuals from a community emergency, such as a train accident, an epidemic, a fire or other internal hospital problem requiring evacuation, or inadequate staffing to safely treat emergency department (ED) patients. Plans should include/address the following:

- Readily available information and disaster preparedness drills
- Activation of the plan, including the individual(s) responsible
- Chain of command
- Facility damage assessment, usually conducted by the facility safety officer
- Hospital/ED capacity to receive individuals
- Triage, including in the community and in the ED
- Transfer protocols for distributing individuals to other facilities
- Staffing, including telephone tree to notify staff to report to facility
- Intra- and interfacility communication and communication with pre-hospital EMS personnel
- Supplies on hand and methods to obtain added supplies
- Delineation of receiving and treatment areas

EVACUATION PROCEDURES

Evacuation procedures for disaster response in the hospital setting should be part of the disaster plan for the facility, and the evacuation route should be posted in each unit. Ambulatory patients should be gathered and guided to a safe staging area or to the outside of the building. Protocol should be followed for the evacuation of non-ambulatory patients. Some can be moved in wheelchairs, but others, such as those with ventilators and multiple invasive devices may need to be transferred in their beds if rapid evacuation is necessary. For vertical evacuations (multi-story facilities), evacuation of non-ambulatory patients may depend on the assistance of fire department personnel if elevators cannot be used. If rapid removal is critical (such as with fire), patients can be placed on sheets and slid onto the floor on the sheets and then pulled down the hallway to the stairs, which can be lined with mattresses on one side. The patients (contained in sheet slings) are then slid down the stairs on the mattresses.

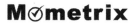

Acute Emergency Situations

FLUID OVERLOAD
SIGNS AND SYMPTOMS

If a patient is suspected to be in **fluid overload**, they should be monitored closely. The most significant sign of fluid overload is increased respiratory distress or crackles in the bases of the lungs. The patient may experience edema in the extremities, puffiness around the eyes, or fluid accumulation (ascites) in the abdomen. As the fluid accumulates, the patient may have unexplained weight gain over a short period of time. A patient in fluid overload may have a bounding pulse, hypertension, or bulging veins. If any of these signs are noticed, the nurse should be notified immediately.

CAUSES

Fluid overload can be **caused** by excessive fluid intake or by acute or chronic medical conditions. Excessive fluid intake can occur if the patient is receiving too much IV fluid or has excessive oral intake. The patient's intake and output balance should be closely monitored to ensure the patient does not continue to take in more fluid than they are putting out. Sodium intake should be monitored as well, as excessive salt intake can increase fluid absorption by the kidneys, resulting in fluid overload. Certain medical conditions, such as heart failure, place the patient at an increased risk of complications due to fluid overload, as the heart may not be able to accommodate an increased amount of fluid. Patients with a history of kidney failure may not be able to effectively compensate for fluid overload and should be closely monitored.

VOMITING IN BED

If the patient begins to **vomit while lying in bed**, the nurse aide should act quickly to make sure the patient does not aspirate on the emesis. The patient should immediately be turned on their side. A basin should be provided to catch any emesis. If there is a suction catheter, use it to clean any vomit from the patient's mouth. After the patient is done vomiting, allow the patient to stay on their side until they have recovered. Rinse the patient's mouth and face with cool water and change the linens if necessary.

SEIZURES

If a patient experiences a **seizure**, the appropriate response is as follows:

- Call for the nurse immediately (emergency light).
- Lower the patient's head (if in bed) or ease the patient onto the floor if in a chair.
- If the patient is in bed, raise bed rails to prevent falls, and pad them with a blanket or other linen to prevent injury.
- Loosen the patient's clothing, especially around the neck.
- Turn the patient onto their side to prevent aspiration and support their head with a pillow or blanket.
- Move furniture and/or other items away from the patient if the patient is on the floor.
- Do not attempt to restrain the patient or to place anything in the patient's mouth.
- Make note of the time the seizure began and ended and the body parts involved in the seizure.
- Ask visitors or others in the vicinity to give the patient privacy.
- Once the seizure has subsided, cover the patient with a blanket and allow the patient to rest until they are alert enough to move.

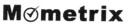

DIABETIC EMERGENCIES

Diabetes mellitus is a chronic condition in which the patient does not produce enough insulin to transport glucose (sugars) to the cells, or the body is not able to effectively utilize insulin. Patients with diabetes mellitus (type 1 or type 2) are at risk for the following **diabetic emergencies**:

- **Hypoglycemia** (excessive insulin intake, resulting in dangerously low blood sugar): The patient may be confused, trembling, with cold and clammy skin and may complain of numbness/tingling and blurred vision. The nurse aide may provide the patient with orange juice, candy, or other sugary food under direction of a licensed nurse as a first line treatment for hypoglycemia.
- **Hyperglycemia** (high blood sugar): The patient may have increased thirst, increased urination, drowsiness, nausea, shortness of breath, and fruity-smelling breath. The patient may require an increased dose of insulin, which requires a doctor's order and nurse administration.
- **Diabetic ketoacidosis** (severely high blood sugar resulting in the breakdown of fat for fuel, which releases ketones that cause acidosis): The patient may experience the signs of hyperglycemia as well as an abnormal pulse (increasing the risk for cardiac arrest) and hyperventilation. These patients require emergency insulin and fluid administration.

In all cases, the nurse aide should immediately call the nurse (using the emergency light if necessary) and remain with the patient.

ACUTE BLEEDING

Acute bleeding (large amounts of bright red blood) may result from injury (such as a fall with large or deep lacerations), rectal bleeding, vaginal bleeding, intracranial bleeding (due to a ruptured artery), severe nosebleed, or a patient's removal of an intravenous or intraarterial catheter. This bleeding can be externally visible, or internal, which is reflected through an acute change in vital signs (decreased blood pressure, increased pulse and respiratory rate, and altered mental status). The nurse aide should remain calm and immediately call for the nurse (using the emergency light if necessary) and should remain with the patient, donning gloves to avoid skin contact with any blood.

- If there is a **bleeding wound**, the location should be elevated and pressure applied to the wound with gauze or clean linen until the nurse arrives.
- If the patient is experiencing an **acute nose bleed**, the nurse aide (or the patient) should apply pressure to the nose by pinching directly above the nostrils. Instruct the patient to lean forward to minimize the risk of aspirating or choking on blood.
- The patient **should not be given any food or drink** and should be **covered to keep warm** and provided reassurance that help is on the way.
- The nurse aide may take the patient's **vital signs** if their hands are free as the patient may go into shock if blood loss is excessive. Signs of shock include pale, cool, and clammy skin, rapid pulse, and low blood pressure.

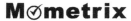

CHEST PAIN

When a patient complains of **chest pain**, the immediate response should be to call a nurse to evaluate and assist the patient (if the pain is severe or the patient is in distress, use the emergency light). The nurse aide should remain with the patient, loosen the patient's clothing (especially around the neck), and measure the patient's pulse and respirations. If equipment is available in the room, the nurse should measure the patient's blood pressure and oxygen saturation level as well. The nurse aide can also gather information if the patient is able to discuss when the pain started, what the pain feels like (dull, aching, sharp, crushing, burning), and exactly where the pain is located. This information is especially valuable in the event the patient experiences a cardiac arrest before the nurse arrives. The nurse aide should avoid giving the patient any food or fluids.

CARDIAC ARREST

Time is of the essence in treating a patient who is found unresponsive. If the patient is unarousable, call for help immediately. Check for breathing by leaning close to the patient's nose and mouth, listening for breath sounds, and watching for the rise and fall of the chest, while palpating the carotid artery (on the side of the neck) to check the patient's pulse. If the patient does not have a pulse, they are experiencing **cardiac arrest**. In this case, if help has not yet arrived, the nurse aide should immediately call for help using the appropriate signal ("Code blue!"), lower the patient's head of bed (if in bed) and prepare the patient for CPR. A backboard can be placed if available and the patient's clothing loosened. If the patient is in a chair, the patient should be eased onto the floor and placed in supine position. Depending on CPR training and protocol, the nurse aide may initiate chest compressions if the patient is positioned appropriately and no nurse is readily available. Compression only CPR is at the rate of 100-120 compressions per minute. If two rescuers are present, the rate is 30 compressions to 2 respirations, starting with compressions. CPR should be performed until the AED arrives at the scene. As soon as the AED is available, the machine should be turned on, and the pads should be attached to the patient's chest per AED instructions. The AED will then analyze the patient's rhythm. While analyzing, nobody should be touching the patient. The machine will then instruct on whether a shock is needed or CPR should be resumed. More often, the nurse aide assists in gathering equipment, such as a crash cart and AED, to support the nurse's resuscitation efforts.

CHOKING

Common indications that a patient is **choking** is the holding of or pointing to the neck with little to no sound being produced. The Heimlich maneuver should only be initiated if the patient is conscious but unable to speak or make noise. The CNA should move behind the patient and wrap his or her arms around them. Make a fist with one hand and place it against the patient's abdomen with the thumb about 2 inches above the umbilicus. Wrap the other hand around the fist. Thrust the fist inward and upward with as much force as possible. Continue to do this until the object has been dislodged from the airway or until the patient loses consciousness. If a patient loses consciousness, their pulse should be assessed. If pulseless, they should be treated for cardiac arrest.

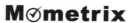

NURSE AIDE RESPONSIBILITIES IN CODE SITUATIONS

In a **code situation**, it is vital for the health care team to work together in order to provide a positive outcome for the patient. Prior to a code, the nurse aide should be aware of their responsibilities. They should know the location of the crash cart in case they are asked to retrieve it and how to activate the code system if they discover a patient who is unresponsive. In a code situation, the nurse aide's primary role will be to obtain any necessary equipment. If they have CPR certification, the nurse aide may also provide relief CPR. It is important that the nurse aide listen to any instructions provided to them. If the room is crowded, the nurse aide should leave the room but remain near the door so that he or she can hear any instructions or needs to attend to.

SAFETY PRECAUTIONS DURING OXYGEN ADMINISTRATION

There are a number of precautions that should be taken to ensure the patient's safety while receiving **oxygen therapy**.

- The patient should be carefully monitored to ensure they are on an appropriate amount of oxygen.
- The patient and family members should be reminded of the facility's no smoking policy, as oxygen is highly flammable.
- Petroleum-based products should not be used while the patient is on oxygen, as these are also highly flammable.
- Care should be taken to make sure the patient does not become entangled in the oxygen tubing.
- Oxygen tanks should be stored in their appropriate holders; an oxygen tank can cause serious harm if it were to be knocked over.

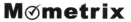

Caring for the Dying Patient

HOSPICE CARE

Hospice care is a series of services that are available to provide end-of-life care for patients with terminal illnesses. Hospice care is typically made available to patients with a life expectancy of six months or less, requiring the sign off of two physicians to confirm this diagnosis. A patient can receive hospice care at home, in a hospital, or in an extended-care setting. The purpose of hospice care is to help the dying patient to pass with dignity, while managing pain and other symptoms and making the patient comfortable. The patient is cared for medically, while receiving spiritual and psychological support. Similar emotional support is provided to family members of the patient.

STAGES OF GRIEF FOR THE DYING PATIENT

When a patient is informed that their condition is terminal and death is inevitable, they typically undergo **five stages of grief**. These stages can occur in any order prior to acceptance of the diagnosis, and the amount of time spent in each stage is dependent upon the patient.

- The first stage is **denial**. The patient is unable or unwilling to accept that they are going to die and often claims that a mistake has been made.
- The next step is **anger**. The patient is unable to deny the illness and reacts with resentment and anger.
- The following step is **bargaining**. The patient attempts to make a deal with a higher power in order to prolong life.
- **Depression** is the next step as the patient realizes that bargaining will not work to undo the situation.
- The final stage is **acceptance** as the patient realizes the situation and begins to make end-of-life preparations.

CARING FOR DYING PATIENT

Patient care should be provided as often as needed for a patient who is dying. The patient should be kept clean; if the patient needs to be bathed while the family is in the room, the family should be asked to step out while patient care is being performed. The only exception is if the patient asks certain members to stay or if their culture requires them to be bathed by family members. Oral care should be provided every two hours and as needed. If excessive oral secretions build up, the patient's nurse should be notified so the mouth can be suctioned gently. The patient should be turned every two hours unless excessive pain is involved, in which case the patient's comfort should be prioritized. Vital signs are typically not ordered for routine monitoring on a patient who is dying.

PRIORITIES

If a patient is actively dying, there are a number of **priorities** that should be kept in mind while caring for the patient. The patient should be kept as free of pain as possible. If the patient complains of pain, notify the nurse immediately so that the patient can be medicated appropriately. The patient should also be kept as comfortable as possible. Allow them to eat and drink what they wish. Listen to the patient's concerns and provide emotional support to both the patient and the family. Allow the family to remain at bedside. Keep in mind that, even if the patient appears to be comatose, the sense of hearing is the last sense to fade prior to death. The nurse aid should encourage the family to continue to talk to the patient, and the nurse aid should take care with his or her own words.

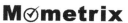

FEEDING

A dying patient is not taking in **adequate nutrition**, so their metabolism changes and energy declines. When this happens, the patient will have less awake time, which can cause the family concern. Food is often associated with comfort. The family's inability to provide this comfort for their loved one can be a source of distress. The CNA or nurse can assist the family by educating them on the problems the patient may experience by consuming more than desired at this point. The dying patient's altered metabolism means that their body is unable to handle nutrients in a normal way. Excess food will cause an increase in respiratory and gastric secretions that can result in dyspnea, abdominal distention, pain, and peripheral edema. All of these conditions put the patient at risk for infection, skin breakdown and pain.

PROVIDING FLUIDS

Most actively dying patients are **dehydrated** because they are no longer consuming adequate food and fluids, but there is little discomfort associated with this state. Family should be informed that dehydration helps reduce nausea, vomiting, and edema for end-stage patients. The most common complaint is dry lips, nasal membranes, and mouth. Oral and nasal drying often results from mouth breathing, medication side effects (e.g., antihistamines), and supplementary oxygen delivered by mask or nasal cannula. The family may wish to provide the patient with fluids to drink as a way to relieve suffering and offer comfort. However, the result could be to add to the patient's distress by increasing respiratory and gastrointestinal secretions as food would. Increased secretions lead to dyspnea, abdominal pain and distention, and peripheral edema. A bloated patient is at risk for skin breakdown, infection, and pain. The nurse aide should cleanse the patient's mouth and lips frequently with cool water or protective gel to help them retain moisture and to ease the discomfort without creating more problems.

SIGNS AND SYMPTOMS OF IMPENDING DEATH

When **death is imminent**, the patient will experience a significant change in vital signs. The heart rate will become slow and irregular, and the pulse will feel weak when palpated. The patient's respiratory rhythm will become shallower, with the breaths becoming infrequent and/or irregular. The breathing may take on a rattling quality that results from mucous in the respiratory tract; this is referred to as a "death rattle." Blood pressure and temperature will decrease. As a result of the diminished vital signs, the patient will become unarousable. Death typically occurs within minutes after the blood pressure is lost.

PROVIDING COMFORT MEASURES AND DIGNITY AS DEATH APPROACHES

The nurse aide should prepare family and friends for the changes they will see as the patient nears death and provide guidance in **comfort measures** for the dying patient:

- Ensure pain is managed adequately, including medications, such as analgesics and muscle relaxants (if the patient is having muscle spasms), and complementary therapies, such as massage, Reiki, and music therapy.
- Provide mouth care with premoistened swabs.
- Gently wash and moisturize the patient's skin with a warm cloth if the patient is cold and cool cloth if feverish.
- Talk softly to the patient even if the patient appears to be in a coma and nonresponsive.
- Accept and do not challenge the patient if they appear to be seeing or communicating with deceased loved ones.
- Utilize video chat technology to allow family/friends who are not present to participate.

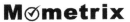

After the patient has died, some people will want to spend time sitting with the body and may want to participate in washing and dressing the body, and the nurse aide should respect these wishes.

RIGOR MORTIS

Rigor mortis is the stiffening of muscles that occurs after death, making the limbs very difficult to move. It typically occurs within a few hours after death and can last up to 72 hours after the time of death. It results from the breaking down of muscle tissue, which releases chemicals within the muscle that cause them to stiffen. **Rigor mortis** is significant because the patient's body can get "stuck" if left in a certain position after death. For this reason, it is important to place the patient in a supine position as soon as possible after death. Certain facility policies call for loosely binding the patient's hands during postmortem care to prevent the limbs from freezing in unusual positions.

ALGOR MORTIS

Normal body temperature is about 37 °C (98.6 °F), but when body functions cease at death, **algor mortis** ("cold death"), a gradual decrease in body temperature, begins within approximately one hour. The body starts to cool by about 1 °C (1.8 °F) every hour until it reaches **ambient temperature**. The exterior surface temperature cools more rapidly than the internal temperature, and the overall rate of cooling may vary depending on the patient's internal temperature at the time of death, the ambient temperature of the environment, the patient's size (muscle mass, fat), and the presence and thickness of clothing or blankets. High temperatures (internal or external) slow the cooling process. As the body cools, the skin loses elasticity and takes on a waxy appearance. This stage of the process of death ends when the temperature begins to rise again as part of **decomposition**, generally within 24 hours.

POSTMORTEM CARE

Postmortem care is the process of preparing a body to be taken to the morgue. The nurse aide should make sure to treat the body with the utmost respect. Ensure privacy by pulling the curtain, then wash the hands and don a pair of gloves. If the patient has dentures, place them in the patient's mouth. Close the patient's eyes. Wash the body as if performing a complete bed bath before dressing the patient in a clean gown. Place a pad over the perineal area. Remove any tubes and lines, and place a dressing over the line insertion sites to prevent oozing. If the facility policy calls for it, shroud the body in a sheet. Place the body in a plastic body bag by tucking it underneath in a manner similar to changing an occupied bed. Label the patient per protocol, which generally includes placing a patient label on the patient's toe and an additional label on the outside of the body bag. Close the bag, tie the zippers shut, and slide the body onto a morgue cart using the assistance of one other colleague.

PROVIDING SUPPORT TO GRIEVING FAMILY MEMBERS

If the family is not present when the patient dies, the nurse aide should make an effort to make the body look presentable prior to the arrival of the family. The body should be placed in a supine position and covered with a blanket up to the chest. If necessary, a clean gown should be placed on the body. The family should be given as much time as they need to view the body. The nurse aide should make an effort to offer comfort to the family, listening to them and providing emotional support where needed. The nurse aide should offer the family anything they might need, such as tissues or water. While viewing the body, the family should be afforded privacy by closing the curtain and shutting the door.

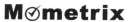

Therapeutic and Technical Procedures

MEASURING INTAKE AND OUTPUT

Intake and output (I&O) is an important indicator of fluid balance. Intake is calculated by measuring all of the fluid the patient takes in orally and intravenously. Output is calculated by measuring all of the fluid the patient excretes, including urine, stool, and emesis. All measurements should be recorded in milliliters (mL). Calculating I&O over a period of a few days can give an indication of the patient's fluid status. Ideally, intake should equal output. If intake exceeds output, then the patient may be fluid overloaded. If output exceeds intake, the patient may be dehydrated.

INTAKE

In order to measure a patient's intake, the nurse aide must measure any liquids the patient takes in over a 24-hour period. This includes any water, milk, and juice the patient might drink, as well as any foods that melt at room temperature, such as ice cream, pudding, or jello. While measuring intake, the nurse aide should also include any tube feeding or any fluid that is used to flush a nasogastric tube. If the patient is receiving IV therapy, all IV fluids and medications suspended in IV fluid should be included in the patient's total intake. IV intake should also include any IV fluids that the patient received during surgery. Intake should be calculated in milliliters (mL) and added up over a 24-hour period. That total should then be reported to the nurse.

OUTPUT

Output measures the amount of fluid the patient excretes during a 24-hour period. All urine should be measured prior to being discarded. The amount of liquid stool in a bedpan should be estimated prior to being discarded. If the patient has a nasogastric tube to wall suction, the nurse aide should note how much drainage the patient has had out of the tube. The cannister should be marked with time and date to allow for accurate measurement from one shift to the next. If the patient has a wound that is hooked to suction, note how much blood has been removed from the wound. If the patient is having drainage out of a wound that is not to suction, the nurse aide should note how many times the dressing needs to be changed. Estimated blood loss from surgery should also be included as output. Add all secretions over a 24-hour period, and make a note of it on the patient's chart.

CALCULATION

After intake and output have been calculated over a 24-hour period, the two numbers should be compared. Ideally, intake should equal output as this indicates an equal fluid balance. Excessive intake puts the patient at a risk for fluid overload, while excessive output puts the patient at risk for dehydration. After comparing intake and output over a 24-hour period, the nurse aide should compare intake and output over the past few days. This gives a better indication of the patient's ongoing fluid status. For example, a high intake on one day may be compensated on the following day with a high output, placing the patient's fluid balance at an equal level.

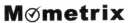

MEASURING HEIGHT AND WEIGHT

USING AN UPRIGHT SCALE

An **upright scale** can be used to measure the patient's height and weight if they have the strength to stand on the scale. The process for using an upright scale is as follows:

1. Prior to measuring a patient's height and weight, the nurse aide should wash hands, greet the patient, and explain what is going to be done.
2. Confirm the patient's identity using two patient identifiers.
3. Assist the patient to a standing position, and guide them to the upright scale.
4. Instruct the patient to stand on the scale, facing away from the scale.
5. Lower the height rod until it rests on top of the patient's head. Make a note of the height.
6. Assist the patient in turning until they are facing the scale.
7. Move the weights on the scale until the bar is balanced or wait for the digital scale to settle on a weight; make a note of the patient's weight.
8. Assist the patient back to the chair or bed, and position them for comfort.
9. Wash the hands.

WHILE THE PATIENT IS LYING IN BED

A patient who is bed bound will need to have their height and weight measured while in bed. There are two methods to **measure a patient's weight in bed**: Using a bed scale pad, or using the weighing system embedded in the bed's technology.

To use a **bed scale pad**, first verify the patient's identity using two patient identifiers, then follow the below process:

1. Obtain assistance from a colleague. Roll the patient onto the bed scale pad.
2. Weigh the patient using the bed scale, and make a note of the patient's weight.
3. Remove the bed scale pad.

To use the **embedded scale in the bed**, it is first important to ensure the bed was zeroed prior to the patient's arrival. This is a way of taking the weight of all of the elements on the bed (mattress, sheets, etc.) into the system so that it is able to then calculate the weight of the patient and subtract the weight of these additional elements to provide an accurate reading. This technology allows for the quick and easy daily weight measurements by simply pressing the button on the bed's control pad, and making sure nothing extra is on the bed that wasn't on it when it was zeroed. The most accurate reading is achieved when the bed is in a horizontal position. Record the reading the bed produces and return any personal items to the patient.

To obtain the patient's **height while in bed**, follow the below process:

1. Move the head of the bed into a horizontal position and roll a bath blanket or sheet under the patient. This may require a second person for assistance.
2. Mark the placement of the patient's heels and the top of their head on the bath blanket.
3. Roll the patient off the blanket and measure the distance between the two marks on the pad. Record this as the patient's height.
4. Reposition the patient for comfort and wash hands.

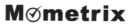

VITAL SIGNS

Vital signs refer to live measurements of an individual's physiology that are most indicative of their health and well-being. Those that are most commonly measured include temperature, pulse, respiration rate, blood pressure, oxygen saturation, and pain level.

- **Temperature** measures the patient's core body temperature.
- **Pulse** (heart rate) measures the number of times the patient's heart beats per minute.
- **Respiration rate** measures the number of times the patient breathes every minute.
- **Blood pressure** is recorded as two numbers. The top number is referred to as the systolic pressure; it measures the pressure within the patient's arteries during contraction of the heart. The bottom number is the diastolic blood pressure; this number reflects the pressure within the arteries while the heart is filling and at rest between each contraction.
- **Oxygen saturation** measures the amount of oxygen in the blood using an electrode that attaches to the finger. This can be measured continuously or intermittently.
- **Pain level** measures the presence or absence of pain. It indicates the severity of that pain according to the patient.

Prior to collecting a patient's vitals, the nurse aide must wash hands, don a pair of gloves, and greet the patient. Explain what is going to be done and verify the patient's identity using two patient identifiers.

TEMPERATURE

AXILLARY TEMPERATURE

To collect an **axillary temperature**, first make sure that the area under the patient's arm is dry. Place a plastic sheath over the temperature probe. Position the thermometer in the axillary area, and instruct the patient to keep his arm down. Leave the thermometer in place until it indicates a reading. Discard the plastic sheath in the trash. Record the temperature, remove the gloves, wash hands, and clean the thermometer prior to using it on another patient.

ORAL TEMPERATURE

To collect an **oral temperature**, first ensure that the patient has not had anything to drink in the past 15 minutes, as this will make a temperature read falsely low. Cover the thermometer with a plastic sheath and place it under the patient's tongue. Instruct the patient to keep the mouth closed and not to talk while the thermometer is obtaining a reading. Wait until the thermometer indicates the temperature has been read. Discard the plastic sheath in the trash. Note the temperature, clean the thermometer, remove the gloves, and wash hands.

RECTAL TEMPERATURE

To collect a **rectal temperature**, first place a plastic cover over the temperature probe. Assist the patient into a side lying position. Apply lubrication to the thermometer, and slide it 1 inch into the patient's rectum. Leave it in place until a temperature reads. Remove the thermometer, inspect it to make sure it is still intact, and discard the plastic sheath. Record the temperature. Position the patient for comfort. Clean the thermometer, remove the gloves, and wash hands.

INDICATIONS OF ABNORMAL TEMPERATURE

A person's core body temperature is closely regulated to ensure an optimum environment for the complex chemical reactions within the body. The normal temperature range for an adult patient is 97-99 °F (36.1-37.2 °C). A low core body temperature may indicate the onset of an infection. The patient's temperature may also be low after coming from a cold environment, such as the operating room. The primary cause for an elevated temperature (fever) is infection. Because a fever is the

65

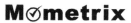

result of the immune system mounting a defense against an infection, it may not be necessary to treat the fever unless the temperature goes above 101.5 °F (38.6 °C).

PULSE
PERIPHERAL PULSE

To measure the peripheral pulse, take the patient's hand and slide the index and middle finger along the thumb, up to the hollow of the wrist. Apply gentle pressure until the pulse can be felt. This is the radial artery and is also referred to as a radial pulse. If the patient's heart rate is regular, count the number of beats for 30 seconds and multiply that number by two. If the patient's heart rate is irregular, count the number of beats for a full minute. Record the number in the patient's chart and wash hands.

APICAL PULSE

An apical pulse measures the number of times the heart beats every minute by auscultating at the apex of the heart. Place the bell of the stethoscope against the patient's left chest and locate the area in which the pulse is the loudest. If the patient's heart rate is regular, count the number of beats for 30 seconds and multiply by two. If the patient's heart rate is irregular, count the number of beats for a full minute. Record the patient's pulse, clean the stethoscope, and wash hands.

INDICATIONS OF ABNORMAL PULSE

The normal pulse range for an adult is 60-100 beats per minute. Patients may have a low heart rate if they are physically fit or resting/sleeping. Some medications may also decrease the patient's heart rate. An elevated heart rate may be the result of exercise, stress, drugs, or caffeine. Certain medications may also elevate the patient's heart rate. If the patient has an elevated temperature or an infection, the heart rate will be elevated. An elevated heart rate can also be the result of uncontrolled bleeding and/or low blood pressure (hypotension) as a compensatory mechanism.

RESPIRATION RATE
MEASURING RESPIRATIONS

Measuring respirations is done to assess the number of times per minute the patient breathes. Typically, when a person is made aware of their breathing, they do not breathe deeply or regularly. For that reason, the nurse aide should not inform the patient when measuring the respiration rate, as it will make them aware of their breathing and may produce an inaccurate result. The ideal time to measure the patient's respiration rate is immediately after checking the patient's pulse. Keep the finger on the patient's wrist so the patient believes their pulse is still being measured, but count the number of times the patient breathes, counting one rise and fall of the chest wall as one respiration. Count the number of breaths for one minute, noting the depth of the breath and any use of accessory muscles. Record the respiratory rate on the patient's chart and wash hands.

INDICATIONS OF ABNORMAL RESPIRATIONS

The normal range for respiration rate is 12-20 breaths per minute. A number of factors may affect the rate of the patient's breathing. The patient may breathe more slowly if resting or if they are positioned on their back. Certain narcotics may also depress the respiratory drive, resulting in fewer breaths per minute. A rapid respiration rate may be caused by increased activity, pain, or stress. An elevated temperature or an infection may cause the patient's respiratory rate to increase. Other conditions, such as respiratory distress, fluid overload, or a heart attack, may also cause an elevated respiratory rate.

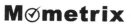

BLOOD PRESSURE
MEASURING BLOOD PRESSURE

To measure a patient's blood pressure, wrap the **blood pressure** cuff around the patient's upper arm about one inch above the antecubital space (bend of the elbow) and place the bell of the stethoscope over the brachial artery. Pump the bulb of the blood pressure cuff, inflating the cuff to 150-180 mmHg. Slowly release the pressure, while listening through the stethoscope. Note the pressure at which a pulse is first heard; this is the systolic blood pressure. Continue to listen to the pulse. Note the pressure at which the pulse fades away; this is the patient's diastolic blood pressure. If the reading is excessively high or low, repeat to confirm and measure the reading on the opposite extremity. Record the findings on the patient's chart and wash hands.

MEASURING ORTHOSTATIC BLOOD PRESSURE

Orthostatic hypotension is a condition in which the patient's blood pressure drops as a result of a change in position. This can cause dizziness or lightheadedness after standing, which may lead to falls. To check for orthostatic hypotension, measure the patient's blood pressure while they are lying down. Next, assist the patient into a sitting position and measure the blood pressure again on the same extremity. If the patient is able to stand, assist them into a standing position and measure the blood pressure a third time. If the patient's blood pressure drops by more than 20 mmHg systolic or 10 mmHg diastolic, then they are considered to have orthostatic hypotension. The nurse should be notified immediately.

INDICATIONS OF ABNORMAL BLOOD PRESSURE

The normal systolic blood pressure is 120 mmHg. The normal diastolic blood pressure is 80 mmHg. Hypotension (abnormally low blood pressure) is defined as a systolic blood pressure less than 90 mmHg and/or a diastolic blood pressure less than 60 mmHg. The patient may have a low blood pressure because they are resting or as a result of certain medications. Bleeding, infection, heart failure, or dehydration may also result in hypotension. Hypertension (abnormally high blood pressure) is defined as a systolic blood pressure greater than 140 mmHg and/or diastolic blood pressure greater than 90 mmHg. High blood pressure can be caused by chronic illness (kidney failure, heart disease, or certain neurological disorders), pain, or stress.

OXYGEN SATURATION

Pulse oximetry non-invasively measures a patient's oxyhemoglobin (**oxygen saturation**) level using a small clip-like device with a sensor that measures the oxygen saturation of the site to which it is attached. This is a painless method of monitoring an individual's respiratory status and perfusion over a period of time when attached continuously, or intermittently as part of a physical assessment. Attach the oximeter sensor to one of the patient's first three fingers (index, middle or ring). If the patient's hands are damaged or excessively cold/poorly perfused, use a toe or earlobe. Consider using the forehead, nose, or other parts of the foot only as a last resort. Normal range should fall between 95% and 100%, although patients with certain conditions, such as COPD, may have a chronically lower saturation. If a patient's oxygen saturation falls below normal range persistently, the nurse aide must inform the nurse immediately, as it may indicate that the patient is hypoxic (not getting enough oxygen). Many pulse oximeters also measure the patient's heart rate at the same time. A pulse oximeter is not accurate if the patient is very anemic, has poor circulation (due to being cold or having vascular abnormalities), is edematous, moves a lot, or wears artificial nails or very dark nail polish.

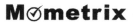

PAIN LEVEL
AREAS ADDRESSED WHEN ASSESSING PAIN

Information concerning a patient's pain can be gathered from a variety of sources, including observations, interviews with the patient and family, medical records, and observations of other health care providers. However, it is important to remember that each patient's pain is **subjective** and **personal**. Pain is defined as whatever the patient says it is. Having the patient give parameters of quality, location, duration, speed of onset, and intensity can all be beneficial in the health care team forming a treatment plan based on the patient's needs. Pain is also influenced by psychological, social, and spiritual factors. Vital signs can be helpful in further defining a patient's pain parameters.

PHYSICAL SIGNS OF PAIN

The best assessment of the patient's pain is **the patient's own report**. All other information is assessed as supporting this report. However, when this method is restricted or unavailable, **physical signs and symptoms** can help the nurse's assessment capabilities. It is important to be familiar with the patient's **baseline** or resting information to give a clear picture of the changes the body may go through when experiencing significant pain. Systolic blood pressure, heart rate, and respirations may all increase above the patient's normal parameters. Tightness or tension may be felt in major muscle groups. Posturing can also occur: the patient may guard areas of the body, curl themselves up into a fetal position, or hold only certain body portions rigid. Calling out, increased volume in speech, and moaning can also be indicators. Facial expressions, such as flat affect or grimacing, and distraction from their surroundings also indicate a significant increase in stressful stimuli. The nurse aide should make note of things that increase the patient's pain and notify the nurse. The nurse aide should make note of new onset/acute pain as this may indicate an emergency.

UNIDIMENSIONAL TOOLS FOR PAIN ASSESSMENT

Unidimensional tools for pain assessment focus on one aspect only: the patient's level of pain. When collecting the patient's pain level as part of their vital signs, there are various methods the nurse aide can utilize:

- **Visual analog/numeric rating scale**: A 1-10 rating scale presented visually or verbally from which the patient chooses a number to describe the degree of pain the patient is experiencing. 0 represents no pain, 1 very mild pain, and 10 the most severe pain the patient can imagine.
- **Descriptive**: Pain is described in simple terms that a patient can choose from: mild, moderate, or severe. This may be especially helpful for patients from other countries or cultures where the 1-10 scale is not generally used.
- **FACES**: A chart shows a facial expression scale of simple drawings showing faces with different emotions, such as happiness, fear, and pain. Used primarily for children over age 3 and for nonverbal adults, although both a child's and an adult's version are available. A revised version applies numeric values to expressions so that pain can be assessed according to a numeric rating scale as well.

68

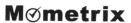

URINE SPECIMEN COLLECTION

COLLECTING URINE SPECIMEN FROM FOLEY CATHETER

When collecting a urine specimen from a catheter bag, care must be taken to ensure bacteria are not introduced into the Foley tubing as this may cause a urinary tract infection. Clamp the catheter tubing 6 inches above the drainage bag, and allow urine to collect in the tubing above it. Thoroughly clean the collection hub with an alcohol swab. Carefully access the collection hub (located attached to the tubing close to the patient) using a Luer-Lok syringe. Collect the desired amount of urine. Transfer the urine from the syringe into the specimen cup, taking care not to touch the cup with the syringe. Tightly close the lid of the specimen cup and place it in a lab specimen bag. Unclamp the catheter tubing. Dispose of the syringe. Remove the gloves and wash hands.

COLLECTING CLEAN-CATCH URINE SPECIMEN

Care must be taken while collecting a urine specimen to make sure that it does not become contaminated during the collection process. A clean-catch urine specimen can be collected from a patient who is able to void. Provide the patient with a sterile specimen cup. Instruct the patient to wash their hands and perineal area thoroughly prior to voiding. The patient should start the stream of urine and urinate for at least 2 seconds before beginning to collect urine in the cup. Don a pair of gloves. Once the patient has acquired a suitable specimen, close the specimen cup tightly and place it in a lab specimen bag. Encourage the patient to wash their hands. The nurse aide should then remove the gloves and wash hands.

STOOL SPECIMEN COLLECTION

A stool specimen is collected from the patient if there is suspicion of an infection or bleeding in the bowels. When the patient needs to have a bowel movement, wash the hands, don a pair of gloves, and explain to the patient what is going to be done. Position a specimen collection hat in the commode to catch stool without catching urine as well. Assist the patient to the bedside commode, provide privacy, and allow them to have a bowel movement. After assisting the patient back to bed, place a small amount of stool into a sterile specimen cup using a tongue depressor or applicator stick and close the lid tightly. Place the specimen cup into a lab collection bag. Dispose of the remaining stool and the hat. Remove the gloves, and wash hands.

SPUTUM SPECIMEN COLLECTION

A sputum specimen is often collected to check for infections in the patient's respiratory tract. To collect a sputum specimen, encourage the patient to cough forcefully to expel sputum from the upper respiratory tract. Instruct the patient to spit the sputum specimen into the cup. If the secretions are thin and clear, it may simply be saliva from the mouth; this is not an adequate specimen. Close the lid of the specimen cup tightly, and place it into a lab specimen bag. Remove the gloves, and wash hands.

OBSERVATIONS DURING INTRAVENOUS THERAPY

An intravenous (IV) line is a small tube that pierces the patient's skin and rests in the vein. It serves as a method of providing the patient with medication and fluids. While receiving **IV therapy**, the patient should be closely monitored to make sure the IV line is in place. If the IV is leaking or oozing at the site, it may be an indication that the hub is not properly connected. If the patient complains of pain from the IV site coupled with warmth, redness, or swelling, it may be a sign that the IV line is no longer in the vein. All of these signs should be reported to the nurse.

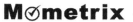

Data Collection and Reporting

CHAIN OF COMMAND ON NURSING UNITS

The chain of command in the nursing unit may vary according to the size, type, and complexity of the facility and unit. Regardless, the usual chain of command is determined by reporting responsibilities.

Role	Responsibilities
Supervisor or manager	This individual is responsible for the management of the unit and the entire staff. They may also be designated as charge nurse or head nurse.
Nurse practitioner or nurse team leader	This individual is responsible for the care of a group of patients and the delegation and supervision of nurses and assistive personnel involved in their care.
RN	This individual is a team member or may serve in the role of team leader or supervising nurse in certain settings. A staff nurse may be assigned specific duties, such as medicating patients or carrying out medical treatments, and may delegate and supervise assistive personnel.
LVN or LPN	This individual usually works under the supervision of an RN and can carry out some medical treatments as well as the delegation and supervision of assistive personnel, depending on the state's scope of practice.
CNA	This individual provides patient care under the supervision of licensed personnel.

OBJECTIVE AND SUBJECTIVE DATA

Objective data refers to information that can be referred to as fact. Objective data is quantifiable, such as vital signs, the patient's weight, or intake and output. Objective data also refers to anything that can be observed by another person. For example, if the patient has flushed cheeks, this is considered to be an objective fact.

Subjective data refers to anything the patient thinks, feels, or reports. The patient may describe their pain, explain that they feel dizzy or nauseous, or that they are having shortness of breath. The patient may also report vomiting or diarrhea that occurred prior to admission. Because these occurred outside of an observational setting, they would be considered subjective data.

CHARTING

PURPOSES

The purpose of charting is to create an accurate log regarding the care given to the patient, as well as the patient's response to the care. Items typically included in the chart are vital signs, intake and output, assessments, and procedure notes. Assessments are typically recorded on preprinted forms; any abnormalities in the patient's assessment are included in the narrative notes. This is referred to as charting by exception. Notes are made in the patient's chart any time a procedure is performed on the patient. Whether or not the nurse aide makes narrative notes in the chart is dependent upon hospital policy.

PRINCIPLES

The nurse aide must consider the following **principles of charting**:

- While writing in the patient's chart, write with only blue or black ink. Do not use a pencil.
- Write legibly, including only objective information. Avoid speculating or becoming overly emotional in the note.
- In paper charting, if an error is made, draw a single line through the erroneous information. Over the erroneous information, write "Error," the reason for the error, and one's initials. Do not scratch out or scribble over the mistake. Do not use correction fluid to cover any errors.
- Do not edit another person's note or write over another person's writing.

LEGAL REQUIREMENTS OF NURSE AIDE DOCUMENTATION

Legal requirements of nurse aide charting include the documentation of:

- **Care activities**: Bathing, skin care, exercises, ambulating, and important conversations
- **Changes in condition**: Vital signs, mental status, urinary and fecal output, skin color, and unusual occurrences

The nurse aide may access only those parts of the patient's records to which the aide is authorized, and all documentation should be factual (rather than opinion-based), accurate (time, amounts, duration), and complete. Documentation should be done throughout the shift rather than simply at the end and as close to the time the care was provided as possible. Documentation should never be done beforehand in anticipation of providing care, as this is illegal and inaccurate.

ROUTINE AND URGENT REPORTING

ROUTINE REPORTING

Routine reporting includes routine daily care, such as bathing, mouth care, toileting, assisting with activities (sitting in chair), and exercising (range of motion) the patient. Routine reporting involves activities for which no further intervention by the supervising nurse is necessary.

URGENT REPORTING

Urgent reporting includes changes in patient's condition that may indicate a need for evaluation or treatment, such as increased pain, evidence of bleeding, and injuries. If the patient is restrained (according to physician's orders), the patient's status must be reported to the supervising nurse. All other special circumstances must be reported immediately. This includes falls, changes in skin condition, patient complaints, suicidal ideation, and difficult or dangerous behavior, such as patient tampering with equipment, discovery of alcohol or pills in patient's possession, patient's failing to comply with diet, and patient's refusal to cooperate with care activities.

DATA TO REPORT IF PROBLEMS ARE NOTED

If a change in the patient's status has occurred, the nurse aide should notify the patient's nurse immediately. The information should be reported in a succinct manner. The patient's name, as well as the room number and the bed number, should be included in the report. The nature of the problem should be explained, including the time of onset. The nurse aide should report any observations that accompany the problem. For example, if the patient developed confusion two hours ago, the nurse aide should include the manner in which the patient is confused.

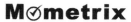

INCIDENT REPORTING

LEGAL OBLIGATION TO REPORT INCIDENTS AND OBSERVATIONS TO LICENSED NURSE

The nurse aide has a legal obligation to immediately report incidents and observations of concern to a licensed nurse, including anything for which the organization may be liable. Incidents usually involve some type of injury or potential for injury (such as a needlestick injury that may result in later infection), and all incidents (whether injury is observed or not) must be reported. The incident report is initiated by the staff member who is involved in or observed the incident but must be reviewed by a supervisor before submission. Incidents may involve:

- **Staff members**: Can include incidents involving the self (needlestick injury, fall, back injury) or others (abuse of patient, administration of treatment to wrong patient, dropping patient)
- **Visitors**: Can include tripping, falling, any type of injury, abusive actions toward patients or staff, and complaints
- **Patients**: Usually involve some problem with the provision of care (wrong treatment), abuse, or accidental injury, such as from falls and restraints

ELEMENTS INCLUDED IN INCIDENT REPORTING

The **elements** that must be included in an incident report are as follows:

- **Name**: The name of the person who is directly involved in or responsible for the incident must be included as well as those affected by the incident and those witnessing the incident.
- **Other identifying information**: Information must be provided so that injured parties and witnesses can be identified and contacted. This includes their birth dates and genders as well as their addresses and telephone numbers.
- **Time, date, and location**: The exact time, date, and location of the incident must be carefully documented. If the time of the incident is not known (such as when a patient is found on the floor), the time the incident was discovered and the last time the person was observed should be documented.
- **Narrative**: A description of what happened and any actions taken at the time (such as lifting a patient) or as a result of the action (transport to x-ray department) must be documented.

WITNESSING A HEALTH CARE PROVIDER BEHAVING NEGLIGENTLY

The nurse aide should be observant for any signs of **negligence** in the health care facility. Negligence can include failing to perform important tasks, such as turning or ambulating, or performing patient care activities in a manner that is unsafe. If the nurse aide sees another member of the health care team behaving in a way that is negligent, they should report that behavior to the charge nurse. If it is the charge nurse who is behaving negligently, the nurse aide should utilize the proper chain of command to make sure the behavior is addressed. Nurse aides should not try to confront negligent coworkers on their own.

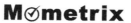

Restorative Skills

BACKRUB PROCEDURE

Providing a patient with a backrub induces relaxation and comfort, critical elements in the restorative process. The process is as follows:

1. Prior to giving a backrub, wash the hands, greet the patient, and explain what is going to be done.
2. Ensure that privacy is provided and don a pair of gloves.
3. If necessary, wash the patient's back with warm water and dry it completely.
4. Warm the lotion in the basin of water and apply a small amount of lotion to the hands.
5. Begin the backrub at the small of the patient's back and work one's way toward the shoulders using long, firm strokes. Use a circular motion when rubbing over bony areas to prevent irritating the skin.
6. While performing the backrub, carefully observe the patient's skin for any signs of breakdown.
7. After the back rub has been completed, position the patient for comfort and wash hands.

SELF-CARE PROGRAM

The purpose of a **self-care program** is to teach the patient how to provide self-care after a long hospitalization or a debilitating illness. The focus of a self-care program may vary depending on the patient's areas of weakness. For example, a patient who has had a stroke and has weakness on one side of the body must be taught how to perform self-care activities safely and effectively. Self-care programs may include physical therapy, occupational therapy, and nutritional therapy. The patient may also receive assistance with medication management, food preparation, and other activities necessary to live within the community.

RESTORATIVE CARE

Restorative care is given to an elderly patient to prepare them for meeting self-care needs after discharge. It is typically provided to patients who have been in the hospital for an extended period of time, such as after breaking a bone or emergent surgery. The type of activities provided during restorative care depends upon individual patient needs. Restorative care commonly focuses upon activities of daily living, including physical therapy, nutrition therapy, and occupational therapy. Emotional support is also provided to the patient to help treat the anxiety and depression that typically accompanies an extended hospital stay.

HOME HEALTH CARE

Home health care is a service provided to patients who are healthy enough to go home but still require the services of a health care provider. The type of home health care provided is dependent upon the patient's needs. Services that may be provided to a patient by a visiting nurse aide may include assisting with daily hygiene, helping the patient to get dressed, cooking meals, feeding the patient, or range of motion exercises. A nurse aide may provide other assistance, such as changing dressings, shopping for food, or taking vital signs.

Psychosocial Care Skills

Emotional and Mental Health Needs

MASLOW'S HIERARCHY OF NEEDS

Abraham Maslow defined human motivation in terms of needs and wants. His **hierarchy of needs** is classically portrayed as a pyramid sitting on its base divided into horizontal layers. He theorized that, as humans fulfill the needs of one layer, their motivation turns to the layer above. He also posited that in order to achieve the higher level of needs, the individual must have the needs of the levels below it met. The layers consist of the following (from bottom to top):

- **Physiological**: The need for air, fluid, food, shelter, warmth, and sleep.
- **Safety**: A safe place to live, a steady job, a society with rules and laws, protection from harm, and insurance or savings for the future.
- **Love/Belonging (Social)**: A network consisting of a significant other, family, friends, co-workers, religion, and community.
- **Esteem and self-respect**: The knowledge that one is a person who is successful and worthy of esteem, attention, status, and admiration.
- **Self-actualization**: The acceptance of one's life, choices, and situation in life and the empathetic acceptance of others, as well as the feeling of independence and the joy of being able to express oneself freely and competently.

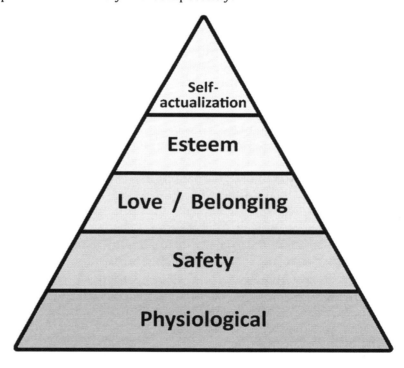

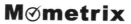

DEFENSE MECHANISMS

Defense mechanisms commonly used by patients include the following:

- **Denial**: Refusing to acknowledge unacceptable realities, such as a terminal illness or inability to carry out activities. Some denial is normal, especially in the beginning, and prevents the patient from becoming overwhelmed with fear or anxiety. However, prolonged denial may prevent the person from seeking treatment or from dealing with feelings.
- **Withdrawal**: Failing to show interest in people or activities and refusing to participate. This is often an indication that the patient is becoming increasingly depressed. Withdrawal is sometimes a protective mechanism to help the patient avoid confronting concerns, such as limited autonomy.
- **Projection**: Accusing others of mistakes, thoughts, or actions that the patient has experienced but feels are unacceptable. This helps the patient to protect his or her self-image.
- **Blaming**: Stating that others are responsible for patient actions in order to protect the self from the response.

ORIENTING A NEW PATIENT TO THE FACILITY

There are a number of methods that a nurse aide can use to **orient a patient to a new facility**. If the patient is only there for a short stay, it may only be necessary to orient them to their room. This includes orienting the patient to the bed controls, call light, and any continuous equipment they may be using, such as telemetry equipment or pulse oximetry. The patient should also be given any necessary information regarding unit policies and visiting hours. If the patient is expected to stay for a long period of time, such as at an extended-care facility, they should also be given a brief tour of the unit. If the facility allows it, the patient may benefit from being introduced to other ambulatory patients.

EMOTIONALLY SUPPORTING PATIENTS

Most patients need some degree of **emotional support** because of the stress of illness and discomfort. The first step in providing emotional support to a patient is to observe carefully and listen attentively. Patients who seem withdrawn or show little interest in activities may be showing signs of depression. The nurse aide should encourage the patient to make decisions about those things within the patient's control, such as food, clothing choices, and times of activities. The nurse aide should provide positive reinforcement ("You did well," or "You are getting stronger") when possible and take time to visit with the patient, especially those patients with no or few visitors. When patients express negative feelings, such as "I hate being sick," the nurse aide should reassure the patient by showing empathy, "I understand how you feel." The nurse aide should use body language (look directly at the patient, smile, nod) to show interest and concern.

ASSISTING PATIENTS IN COPING WITH LOSSES AND ADJUSTMENTS TO NURSING HOME PLACEMENT

Intervention strategies to assist the patient in coping with losses and adjustments to nursing home placement include the following:

- **Control**: The nurse aide should provide the patients with as many opportunities as possible to exercise control, asking their opinions and giving them options whenever possible ("Do you want to walk before or after lunch?").
- **Autonomy**: Autonomy is the patient's ability to act or make decisions based on their personal knowledge and experience. Patients should understand that they have the right to make decisions about their care. If the nursing home allows a private space for belongings (clothing, pictures), the nurse aid should ask the patients how and where they would like their belongings to be placed.
- **Privacy**: The nurse aide should be sure to pull bed curtains and shut doors when working with patients and avoid exposing the patients unnecessarily. Additionally, the nurse aide should speak privately to the patients when discussing personal issues, such as toileting.

DEPRESSION

Depression is a disorder in which the patient experiences a consistently low mood, coupled with feelings of worthlessness, sadness, or self-loathing. The patient may experience insomnia (inability to sleep) or hypersomnia (sleeping excessively). The patient may also complain of digestive difficulties or frequent headaches. Severe cases of depression may result in increased forgetfulness or hallucinations. Depression can be caused by a number of physical, psychological, or sociological factors. Physical characteristics, such as a small hippocampus of the brain, may lead to the onset of depression. Depression may also be brought on by life-altering illnesses, such as Parkinson's disease, heart attack, or stroke. Tragic life events and the inability to effectively cope with them may also lead to an onset of depression.

NEUROLOGICAL DISORDERS
ALZHEIMER'S DISEASE

Alzheimer's disease is a degenerative disorder of the brain. It is the most common cause of dementia. It typically affects people 65 years of age and older, though early onset Alzheimer's disease can occur. The cause of Alzheimer's disease is unknown. Initial symptoms of Alzheimer's disease include loss of short-term memory or forgetfulness. As the disease progresses, the patient experiences increasing confusion and aggression, while losing long-term memory, language skills, and other cognitive functions. Death typically results from breakdown of bodily functions. Though Alzheimer's disease is incurable, management of the disease is the key to an extended life expectancy after diagnosis.

DEMENTIA

Dementia is a term used to describe any cognitive dysfunction that may occur as a result of long-term illness, such as Alzheimer's disease, depression, and cerebral vascular accident. Dementia encompasses any resulting difficulties in memory, language, or problem-solving abilities. The patient is usually considered to be demented after six months of cognitive dysfunction; cognitive dysfunction that has occurred for less than six months is typically referred to as delirium. Dementia may be curable, depending upon the cause. If the patient starts showing any signs of confusion, it should be reported to the nurse immediately.

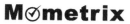

IRREVERSIBLE DEMENTIA

Multi-infarct dementia is the second most common cause of **irreversible** cognitive dysfunction (with Alzheimer's disease being the first). It is caused by tissue damage that occurs when atherosclerotic plaque on the vessel wall breaks off and migrates to another part of the brain, where it creates a blockage. Because the brain tissue cannot get an adequate supply of blood flow, brain tissue in the area of the blockage dies from hypoxia. Though the blockages can be treated, cognitive function does not return after treatment. Huntington's disease is the degeneration of certain types of brain cells. Dementia often develops in the late stages of this disease.

REVERSIBLE DEMENTIA

There are a number of diseases and disorders that result in the onset of dementia. The most common cause of reversible dementia is infection of the brain, such as meningitis or encephalitis. Both the infection and the resulting dementia typically **resolve** after treatment with antibiotics. Disorders that cause undue pressure on the brain, such as head injuries, hydrocephalus, and brain tumors, can cause dementia. There are treatments available to treat the increased pressure, and the dementia diminishes after the pressure has been relieved. Disorders that affect other body systems, such as liver disease, kidney disease, or pancreatic disease, can cause dementia by upsetting the delicate chemical balance within the body. In order to restore the patient's previous mental state, the chemical balance in the body must be restored.

SUNDOWNER'S SYNDROME

Sundowner's syndrome is a condition in which patients become increasingly confused in the late afternoon or early evening. It is most commonly seen in patients with a history of Alzheimer's disease or dementia; however, it can occur in patients who do not have a history of dementia. Though a number of theories exist as to why Sundowner's syndrome occurs, the actual cause is unknown. Patients who are suffering from Sundowner's syndrome may experience worsening confusion, restlessness, or agitation. Some patients may experience hallucinations or wandering as part of Sundowner's syndrome.

STEPS TO ALLEVIATE SYMPTOMS

There are a number of steps a nurse aide can take to decrease the severity of Sundowner's syndrome. In the morning, the nurse aide should open the curtains and blinds and allow the patient to see outside to reorient them to time of day. Encourage exercise during the day. Plan all strenuous activities for the morning so that there is an adequate amount of time to relax prior to bedtime. Do not allow the patient to sleep during the day as this will make it difficult to sleep during the night. Plan a few relaxing activities before bed, such as therapeutic massage or quiet reading time. These activities should be performed at the same time every night to establish a routine. When it is time to sleep, darken the room as much as possible to further reinforce time of day.

PARKINSON'S DISEASE

Parkinson's disease is a disorder that results in degeneration of the nervous system. It causes a decline in speech and motor skills and may cause a decline in cognitive function. Typical signs of Parkinson's disease include tremulousness, a shuffling gait, difficulty turning, difficulty speaking or swallowing, and a mask-like face. Parkinson's disease may also result in short-term memory loss and dementia in advanced cases. In most cases, the cause of Parkinson's disease is unknown, though in some cases the cause may be genetic or a result of a history of head trauma. Treatment includes medication management, management of symptoms, and surgery.

CARING FOR THE CONFUSED PATIENT

Confusion that develops in the hospital or extended-care facility is typically a symptom of a physiological problem. If the nurse aide notices confusion in a patient who was previously oriented, the nurse should be notified immediately. The nurse aide should try to find out what the patient's normal orientation was prior to entering the hospital; this can be done by reviewing records and talking to family members. The nurse aide should be observant for any signs of the physiological problem that may be causing the confusion. For example, cloudy urine may indicate a urinary tract infection, which could result in confusion in the elderly. Until the cause of the confusion is determined, the nurse aide should provide a safe, non-threatening environment while attempting to reorient the patient to the surroundings.

REALITY ORIENTATION

Reality orientation is a set of activities that are performed with a confused patient in an attempt to reorient them to their environment. The first step of reality orientation is to approach the patient in a friendly, non-threatening manner. While interacting with the patient, the nurse aide should provide verbal reminders regarding time and place. The nurse aide should provide the patient with physical reminders of the surroundings, such as writing the date on a whiteboard within the patient's visual field or showing the patient where a clock can be located.

CARING FOR THE AGITATED PATIENT

When a patient becomes **agitated**, the key is to remain calm. Gently reorient the patient to their surroundings and situation. Speak softly but clearly and attempt to learn what it is that is causing the patient to become agitated. While talking to the patient, assume a non-threatening posture. If possible, enlist the aid of family members to calm the patient down. If all of these measures fail and the patient is behaving in a way that may cause harm to the patient or to other people, restraints may be required.

SAFETY AND COMFORT OF PATIENTS WITH PSYCHOLOGICAL IMPAIRMENTS

Psychological impairments may result from psychiatric disease (schizophrenia, bipolar disorder, depression), physical disease (brain tumor, encephalitis, Parkinson's, stroke), or anxiety. Patients with psychological impairments often have difficulty managing ADLs and may have poor social skills, which may interfere with their ability to interact with others or make their needs known. Special considerations for **patient safety and comfort** may include the following:

- Utilizing a locked facility or wander management system
- Assisting patient with ADLs and basic hygiene
- Noting changes in behavior, attitude, or emotional state and reporting these to the nurse
- Monitoring intake and output to ensure that the diet is adequate and nutritious
- Utilizing any prescribed safety precautions at all times
- Ensuring no dangerous items (knives, scissors) are within access of patients who may be violent or self-harm
- Anticipating patient needs and responding appropriately
- Engaging with the patient and encouraging interactions
- Reassuring the frightened or anxious patient

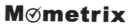

AGE-RELATED NEEDS
OBSERVATIONS WHILE INTERACTING WITH ELDERLY PATIENTS

While interacting with an elderly patient, the nurse aide must be **vigilant to observe** any changes in the patient's mental status. Check to see if the patient is alert or if they appear to be difficult to awaken. Assess the patient for any signs of confusion, such as disorientation to place or time. Make a note of any changes, such as increased weakness, slurring of speech, or the inability to follow commands. If the patient shows any of these signs, the nurse should be notified immediately as these may indicate severe physical or neurological problems.

MENTAL CHANGES INVOLVED IN AGING

Cognitive impairment in the elderly becomes noticeable for adults as young as 60 years of age, though the rate of decline varies depending on the individual. As a person ages, they typically experience a mild decline in the ability to retrieve words and name common objects. Memory also tends to decline as a person ages. The ability to encode new information declines, typically as a result of a decline in sensory abilities. Short-term memory may also decline, though significant changes in long-term memory are typically not seen until about 70-80 years of age. The rate of memory decline can be stemmed using memory exercises and problem-solving skills.

CHARACTERISTICS OF ABUSE

Abuse is any sort of action that results in the physical harm, mental harm, or death of the patient. It is a criminal act and most typically results in imprisonment. Abusive actions can be deliberate or can be the result of negligence. Abuse can take a number of forms, including physical, psychological, verbal, sexual, or financial. Abuse can be subtle and some victims of abuse may be reluctant to come forward. The nurse aide should be vigilant for any signs of abuse and report any findings to the charge nurse immediately.

PSYCHOLOGICAL ABUSE

Psychological or emotional abuse occurs when a person uses psychological attacks in order to intimidate or humiliate another person. It is typically done in order to coerce the victim into doing something that they do not want to do. Psychological abuse can include teasing, threatening harm, or abandonment. Psychological abuse can be difficult to identify because it does not necessarily leave physical marks. A person who has been psychologically abused may show vague symptoms, such as chronic depression, anxiety, anger, or posttraumatic stress disorder. In many cases, other types of abuse accompany psychological abuse.

FINANCIAL ABUSE

Financial abuse occurs when a person takes the money and belongings of another person. The elderly are most commonly the victims of financial abuse. Forms of financial abuse include forcing a person to sign over property, using monthly disability checks for items other than the elderly person's care, or forging another person's signature. Being observant is the best way to catch financial abuse. It is possible that the patient is being abused financially if the patient lacks basic amenities, such as appropriate clothing or necessary personal items, (e.g., glasses or hearing aids) despite adequate financial assistance.

Copyright © Mometrix Media. You have been licensed one copy of this document for personal use only. Any other reproduction or redistribution is strictly prohibited. All rights reserved. This content is provided for test preparation purposes only and does not imply an endorsement by Mometrix of any particular political, scientific, or religious point of view.

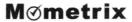

Verbal Abuse

Verbal abuse refers to using words and threats in order to demean or upset another person. **Verbal abuse** includes threatening another person, raising one's voice in anger, or using profanity or derogatory statements toward the other person. It can be difficult to identify a person who is being verbally abused. They may complain of vague symptoms, such as depression, anxiety, anger, or a feeling of hopelessness. In many cases, the victim may blame him or herself for the abuse or may be overcome with hopelessness that the abuse cannot be stopped. Verbal abuse is often accompanied by physical abuse.

Physical Abuse

Physical abuse is the most obvious form of abuse. It occurs when one person deliberately inflicts harm on another person and may be accompanied by verbal, emotional, or sexual abuse. Signs of **physical abuse** include bruising or abrasions with a distinctive shape, such as a fist or foot. Any injuries that do not coincide with the provided explanation should be suspected. For example, a caregiver states that the patient burned himself while cooking. The explanation would be suspect if the burns are in a suspicious place, such as on the inner arm or on the abdomen. If a caregiver refuses to leave the patient's side during an interview or insists upon speaking for the patient, this behavior is also suspicious and should be reported to the nurse.

Sexual Abuse

Sexual abuse is any unwanted sexual behavior directed from one person to another. It includes any sexually suggestive comments or gestures, unwanted touching or fondling, or coercion to perform a sexual act. Additional forms of **sexual abuse** include sexual harassment or behavior that is sexually demeaning. Other forms of abuse may accompany sexual abuse in order to frighten the victim into maintaining silence. Possible signs of sexual abuse include bruising around the perineal area, complaints of abdominal pain, or reoccurring yeast or urinary tract infections. The patient may also exhibit depression or increased anxiety or anger.

Reporting the Abuse of a Patient by Family

It is the obligation of the health care facility to **report any incidences of abuse** to the state in order to protect the victim and remove them from the situation. The nurse aide should be vigilant for any signs of abuse and should report any signs of abuse to the charge nurse. This includes any physical signs of abuse, any statements made by the patient regarding abuse, or any signs of neglect. Once the findings have been reported to the charge nurse, the health care team will determine if any abuse has taken place and notify the proper authorities. The nurse aide should not try to discuss the subject with the victim by herself, and should not attempt to confront or accuse the abuser.

Caregiver Burden and Abuse

In many cases of abuse, the caregiver is responsible for inflicting the abuse on the patient. The abusive behavior may stem from feelings of exhaustion or frustration related to caring for another person. This is often referred to as **caregiver burden**, a feeling that can also be burdensome to nurse aides. Whenever a nurse aide becomes frustrated with a person or situation, they should be removed from the situation as quickly as possible to avoid progressing this caregiver burden to any form of abuse. They should take a moment to try and recognize the source of their frustration. The aide might find it helpful to talk to the charge nurse about their feelings or try to work with a different team of patients on their next shift. If these measures do not work, it would be beneficial for the nurse aide to seek counseling through their job, to protect both oneself and the patients.

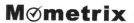

Spiritual and Cultural Needs

INFLUENCING FACTORS ON OUTLOOK IN LONG-TERM CARE

CULTURE

Culture is defined as the behavior and belief systems of a particular group of people. A person's cultural outlook is shaped by ethnicity, gender, and age. It affects their outlook on all things, including health care. It can affect the types of foods patients might eat while sick, their behaviors during illness, and their attitude about death and dying. The patient's cultural beliefs should be taken into account when planning care. If the patient's cultural beliefs are not taken into account, it may increase the patient's stress level, hindering the healing process.

RELIGION

Religion is the set of beliefs that a person has regarding the nature of the universe. The patient's religion may dictate the level of participation in their care, including what treatments they may and may not accept. Religion can also aid in the patient's ability to cope during the recovery period following serious illness or injury. The patient's religious outlook should be taken into account when planning the patient's care. Failure to do so may result in the patient's refusal to participate in the care or withdrawal from the hospital setting altogether.

APPROPRIATE ACTION IF A PATIENT ASKS FOR A PRIEST

During times of illness or injury, it is not uncommon for a patient to request to see a priest or a person of authority within their church. If a patient makes such a request, the nurse aide should notify the charge nurse immediately. The charge nurse will talk with the patient and find out if there is a specific person the patient wishes to see. Most hospitals and extended-care facilities have an on-call clergyperson who can be notified if the patient does not have a specific person to call.

CARING FOR MUSLIM PATIENTS

It is important to ask the **Muslim patient** if they have any specific dietary restrictions. Many strict practicing Muslims will eat only specially slaughtered fish, chicken, and beef. Most Muslims will not eat pork products. Try to avoid handing a Muslim patient anything with the left hand, as that is the hand that is reserved for performing perineal care on oneself. Muslims place a strong emphasis on cleanliness. Many Muslims wish to wash with soap and water after using the bedpan and toilet paper. They should also be provided with fresh water to wash with prior to their prayers. If possible, female patients should be cared for by female nurse aides.

CARING FOR CHRISTIAN PATIENTS

It is important for the nurse aide to ask if the **Christian patient** has any dietary restrictions. Though most Christians do not have dietary restrictions as a result of their faith, some may have self-imposed dietary restrictions. Some Catholic patients may wish to fast during Lent. During their stay, some Catholic or Orthodox Christian patients may choose to receive communion or give confession during their hospitalization. Some patients may request to receive Last Rites if they are critically ill or dying. It is important to notify the charge nurse immediately if the patient requests to see a priest while at the hospital. In many cases, the patient or family will know a priest they would want to call.

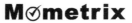

CARING FOR HINDU PATIENTS

It is important for the nurse aide to inquire about any specific dietary needs of the **Hindu patient**. Most Hindus are vegetarian or vegan; even those that do eat meat may refuse to eat beef or pork. After using the bedpan, many Hindu patients want to wash their perineal area using clean water after using toilet paper. The nurse aide should make it available if requested. Some Hindus may prefer to wash in the shower rather than sitting in the bath. Members of the Hindu faith particularly value privacy; if possible, the patient should be cared for by a nurse aide who is of the same gender. Some Hindu patients may prefer to die while lying on the ground to maintain closeness between the individual and Mother Earth. If necessary, a Hindu priest may be called in to perform holy rites for the patient.

CARING FOR JEWISH PATIENTS

Orthodox Jews eat only kosher meat and typically avoid dishes in which milk and meat have been prepared together. Other types of foods that are forbidden include pork products, meat from birds of prey, and shellfish. Most **Jewish patients** prefer to wash their hands and say a brief prayer prior to eating; the nurse aide should provide them with an opportunity to do so. Jewish men may prefer to remain bearded or may choose to shave using an electric razor rather than a razor blade. Jewish patients observe specific practices regarding death. The family will notify their Synagogue of the patient's impending death; if there is no family present, the health care staff should do so. After the death, three members of the family typically wash the body. Burial should take place within 24 hours after dying.

CARING FOR MORMON PATIENTS

Many Mormons follow a set of dietary restrictions put forward in the *Word of Wisdom*. It teaches against the use of stimulants, such as coffee, tea, and other caffeinated beverages. Though most Mormons are not strict vegetarians, they do tend to eat meat sparingly. Some Mormons may wear a special undergarment that should be treated with the utmost privacy. It can be removed for laundering and washing but is otherwise worn at all times. Though Mormons do not have specific rites or rituals regarding a dying patient, the nurse aide should make sure to allow the family to spend as much time as possible with the patient in their final hours. If the patient wears the sacred undergarment, it should be put back on the body after postmortem care has been performed.

CARING FOR BUDDHIST PATIENTS

It is important for a nurse aide to inquire about a **Buddhist patient's** dietary needs on admission as many Buddhist patients are vegetarians or vegans. Many Buddhists fast on specific days, including the days of the New Moon and Full Moon. On fasting days, a Buddhist will only eat at specific times. The nurse aide should collaborate with the patient on these days to ensure they get their meal tray at appropriate times. The type of rituals surrounding death and dying varies depending on the patient's traditions. The patient may request a Buddhist monk or nun to perform chants in order to assist in the patient's passing. If possible, the body should not be touched until 3 to 8 hours after death before preparing the body for death.

Role of the Nurse Aid

Communication

COMPONENTS OF COMMUNICATION

There are five **components** that must be present in order for communication to take place.

Component	Description
Sender	The original source of the message
Message	What the sender is trying to convey
Channel	The means through which the message is being conveyed (typically either verbal or nonverbal)
Receiver	The person who is receiving the message
Feedback	The receiver's response to the original message (roles of sender and receiver may interchange over the course of a conversation)

VERBAL COMMUNICATION

Verbal communication is one way in which people communicate. It encompasses what is said as well as the manner in which it is said. When communicating with the patient, the nurse aide should take into account the patient's language and word choice, as well as the tone of voice and the volume at which the words are spoken. When talking with a patient, it is important for the nurse aide to think carefully about what they say prior to saying it, as words can often be misunderstood. It is also important to ensure that comments are appropriate to the setting and conversation.

NONVERBAL COMMUNICATION

Nonverbal communication is the process of sending messages using methods other than speaking. It can convey emotions and attitudes and can aid in communicating effectively with the patient. A person can communicate nonverbally using gestures, touch, or body language. A nurse aide should closely monitor their own body language to make sure that it does not contradict what they are saying. For example, a nurse aide who talks to the patient while frequently checking their watch is indicating that they are in a hurry. Such body language discourages open communication and should be avoided.

THERAPEUTIC COMMUNICATION

Therapeutic communication is a method of communicating with patients that encourages them to open up and provide information. Because of the level of stress involved in hospitalization, the patient often needs to communicate but is unsure how to initiate conversation with the health care staff. **Therapeutic communication** combines a variety of verbal and nonverbal communication techniques in order to encourage the patient to speak openly. By making note of the patient's body language as well as their words, the nurse aide can interpret the patient's emotional state and communicate with the patient effectively.

83

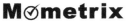

ENCOURAGING COMMUNICATION

There are a number of steps the nurse aide can take in order to **encourage communication** with the patient. First, the nurse aide can ensure the patient is in an environment in which they can communicate freely. If the patient is comfortable, they are more likely to participate in therapeutic conversation. The nurse aide should also ensure the patient's privacy during the conversation. The patient may feel embarrassed about sharing personal information in a public setting. The nurse aide should make an effort to appear unhurried, encouraging the patient to talk by sitting near the patient during the conversation. The nurse aide should also convey interest by facing the patient and maintaining eye contact during the conversation.

SILENCE

Silence can be an effective communication tool because it can convey a number of emotions. While communicating with the patient, **silence** can convey the sentiment of affection. This type of silence is typically accompanied by nonverbal actions, such as a hug or holding the patient's hand. Silence can also be utilized to encourage the patient to give more information. If this is done during a conversation, the patient may continue to talk to fill the silence. Silence can also give the patient time for contemplation. Care must be taken in utilizing silence as a communication tool as it can sometimes be misinterpreted as hostility or rudeness.

ASKING QUESTIONS

Asking questions can be effective in encouraging communication with the patient. There are two types of questions, open-ended and closed-ended.

- **Open-ended questions** encourage the patient to provide added detail about the subject of the conversation, while giving them more control over the conversation. Open-ended questions cannot be answered with one-word responses. "How do you feel about that?" is an example of an open-ended question.
- **Closed-ended questions** can be used to focus the conversation or get it back on track. They are typically used to elicit a one-word answer. An example of a closed-ended question is "Did you eat breakfast today?"

ACTIVE LISTENING

Active listening is the method of listening attentively to the conversation at hand. During a typical conversation, it is common for a person to not devote their full attention to what is being said. They may be thinking of other things or focusing on the work they are trying to do. When a person is **listening actively**, they are not only paying attention to the conversation, but also considering the patient's words and forming an appropriate response that will encourage further conversation. Active listening also takes into account various aspects of nonverbal communication in order to draw the appropriate conclusions from the conversation.

REFLECTING

Reflecting is another method of encouraging the patient to talk about a particular subject. A nurse aide **reflects a statement** by repeating all or part of the patient's original statement back to the patient. For example, the patient says, "I feel so lonely." An appropriate reflective response would be "Lonely?" Another form of reflecting is to make a statement regarding the patient's feelings. For example, the nurse aide may say, "It seems like you are very happy about this." This reflects the patient's emotional state and encourages them to speak openly about what they are thinking and feeling.

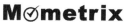

GENERAL LEADS AND RESTATING

A **general lead** is a method used to encourage the patient to continue speaking about a particular subject. Examples of general leads include phrases such as "go on" or "I see." These are effective because they allow the patient to guide the conversation, giving them the opportunity to voice their thoughts and concerns. General leads also indicate that the nurse aide is paying attention to what is being said.

When a nurse aide **restates** something, they rephrase a comment that the patient made earlier in the conversation in order to encourage the patient to elaborate on it. For example, the nurse aide might say, "So you think you have too much equipment on you?" if the patient makes a comment about all of the tubes and wires attached to them.

EMPATHY AND TOUCH

Empathy is the ability to understand what the patient is feeling and to respond appropriately. Acting empathically begins by recognizing any strong emotions the patient might be having. By recognizing these emotions, the nurse aide can give the patient the opportunity to talk about their feelings, as well as provide validation. Acting empathically allows the nurse aide to build trust and understanding with the patient.

Using **touch** is a nonverbal method of communicating with the patient. There are times when words are not enough to provide an adequate amount of comfort. In these times, holding a hand or giving a hug can do more to encourage conversation and provide comfort. The patient's culture must be considered when considering the use of touch, as some cultures may see it as a sign of disrespect.

PROVIDING INFORMATION AND SELF-DISCLOSING

Providing information can be an effective tool in encouraging communication. When the patient is new to the health care facility, they may feel anxious about the unfamiliar surroundings. The nurse aide can help ease anxiety by providing the patient with information that is relevant to their care. However, the nurse aide must be careful not to provide specific information regarding the patient's diagnosis or test and lab results, as this is not within the scope of the nurse aide.

A nurse aide can also encourage communication by **self-disclosing** some information about him or herself in order to ease the patient's discomfort. However, the nurse aide must be careful not to dominate the conversation, as the goal of therapeutic communication is to discover what the patient is thinking and feeling.

COMMUNICATING WITH PATIENT'S FAMILY

Interaction with the **patient's family** can occur frequently during the course of patient care. The nurse aide can confer with the patient's family regarding procedures that are part of the nurse aide's scope of practice. When talking with the family while the patient is in the room, the nurse aide should make an effort to include the patient in the conversation; it is inappropriate to talk about the patient as if he or she is not there. If any family members have a question about the patient's care, they should be referred to the nurse or charge nurse. When the nurse aide is talking to the patient and/or their family, there are a number of ways that they can make sure that what they are saying is clearly communicated. The nurse aide should avoid using medical terminology while talking to the patient as many find it to be confusing. The nurse aide should make an effort to use words that can be understood by the layman. For example, instead of saying hypertension, the nurse aide can be better understood by using the phrase high blood pressure. If a medical term must be used, the nurse aide should define the term for the patient. While talking with the patient, the nurse aide should speak slowly and clearly in a moderate tone of voice.

CALL LIGHTS
ANSWERING THE CALL LIGHT

The **call light** is the way in which a patient notifies the health care staff that they are in need of assistance. It should be answered promptly and courteously. If a call light is going off in a room that is not assigned to the nurse aide, it is appropriate for the nurse aide answer it to find out what the patient needs. If using an intercom, the nurse aide should answer by asking, "May I help you?" If answering the call light personally, the nurse aide should introduce oneself and inquire about the patient's needs. It is not appropriate for the nurse aide to ignore a call light.

FREQUENT USE OF CALL LIGHT

Frequent use of the call bell can occur for a number of reasons. The patient may not understand how to use the call bell or may push the wrong button accidentally. If this happens, a nurse aide can tape a piece of gauze over the button so that the patient can recognize the call button using their fingers. If using this method, it is important to check to make sure the call button can be pushed easily prior to leaving the room. Another reason that a patient may call frequently is that they are lonely. If this is the case, the nurse aide should make an effort to stop in to see the patient as frequently as possible. This may prevent frequent calls "just to chat." One way to prevent frequent use of the call bell is to make sure the patient has all necessary items within reach prior to leaving the room. Also, ask the patient if there is anything else they might need prior to leaving the room.

COMMUNICATION BARRIERS
COMMUNICATION BLOCK

A communication block is a statement or behavior that discourages therapeutic communication. A nurse aide may inadvertently use a communication block if they are hurried or uncomfortable about the conversation at hand. **Common communication blocks** include the use of sarcasm or jokes in order to deflect the situation. The nurse aide may change the subject or may attempt to minimize the problem in order to ease their own discomfort. Offering false assurances or telling the patient how they should feel in a given situation may discourage the patient from communicating with the nurse aide.

COMMUNICATING WITH PATIENTS WHO CANNOT SPEAK ENGLISH

Patients who are unable to speak English may be a challenge to communicate with. Though it is possible to ask a family member to help in translating, many facilities prefer to use an official interpreter when conveying medically related information to the patient. Whether communicating through a family member or an interpreter, the nurse aide should look at the patient and address them while speaking. The aide should speak slowly and clearly, and watch the patient's body language and facial expressions closely as this can help in the communication process. Before the family leaves, the nurse aide should ask them to write down a few common phrases, such as bathroom and water, to help with meeting the patient's needs.

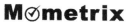

HANDLING INAPPROPRIATE COMMENTS TOWARD STAFF

Some patients may attempt to use sexual innuendo jokingly or as a way to ease their own discomfort. However, such comments are considered to be harassment. Members of the health care staff have a right to work in an environment that is free of harassment. Some may try to diffuse the situation with a joke, but this approach is typically ineffective in halting the abusive behavior. If the patient begins making inappropriate comments, the nurse aide should immediately inform the patient that their comments are unacceptable and will not be tolerated. This should be stated firmly, but politely. If the patient continues the inappropriate behavior, the charge nurse should be notified.

INABILITY TO COMMUNICATE WITH PATIENT

Sometimes the nurse aide may be unable to communicate with the patient despite his or her best efforts. If the patient is intubated or has severe aphasia, they may not be able to effectively communicate their needs. The nurse aide should attempt to figure out what the patient is trying to say by running through a list of common needs, such as being thirsty, hot, cold, or in pain. If the nurse aide cannot decipher what the patient is trying to say, they should tell the patient that they are unable to understand. They should not pretend to understand as this behavior can cause distress for the patient. The inability to communicate often results in frustration on the part of the patient. If this happens, the nurse aide should provide appropriate reassurance and emotional support.

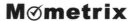

Client Rights

PATIENT'S BILL OF RIGHTS

The Patient's Bill of Rights is a list of rights that the patient can expect to receive while staying in a hospital or an extended-care facility. This list of rights may differ in wording from hospital to hospital but generally contains similar provisions. The Patient's Bill of Rights is typically accompanied by a list of responsibilities that the patient should adhere to in order to ensure their treatment is effective. It is important that the patient be made aware of their rights and responsibilities as soon after admission as possible.

SPECIFIC PATIENT RIGHTS

CONFIDENTIALITY

The patient has the right to **confidentiality**. In other words, they have the right to have their health and health care discussed only by those who are directly responsible for that care. Unless a nurse aide is caring for the patient, they should not review a patient's chart or discuss their case. Furthermore, once the nurse aide is no longer providing care to the patient, they should not access that patient's records. After the patient is transferred to another unit of the hospital, the nurse aide should not access their files. Patient information should be discussed in areas where other people cannot overhear it to prevent laypeople from hearing details about the patient's care.

PRIVACY

Patients have a right to **personal privacy**. The nurse aide should make an effort to protect the patient's privacy by maintaining his dignity during patient care procedures. While bathing the patient or taking him or her off of the bedpan, the curtain or door to the room should be closed to prevent other people from seeing in.

Patients' right to privacy also applies to their health information. Details of a patient's case should only be discussed with the family members that the patient specifies. Many facilities have developed a system involving a privacy code number that is only given to the family members that are to receive information regarding the patient. Unless the family member is able to provide the privacy code number, the nurse aide cannot provide any information to that individual.

INFORMED CONSENT

The idea of informed consent originally came about in reference to experimental treatment. However, it has come to encompass the type of information that should be provided prior to every test, procedure, or treatment. Before signing the consent form, the patient has the right to be informed about all of the risks and benefits involved in the proposed treatment, as well as the risks and benefits involved in refusing the treatment. They should be told which doctors will be involved in their care and what medications they will receive. The doctor should provide this information prior to the procedure, either directly to the patient or to the patient's health care power of attorney. Once received, the patient (or their POA) must sign a consent form stating that they understand all of the required elements. While the nurse aide is not responsible for providing this information or signing as a witness, they can report any lingering questions the patient may have to the nurse because these questions would require the doctor's answers prior to obtaining consent.

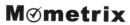

FREEDOM OF CHOICE

The patient's right to freedom of choice works in conjunction with the right of informed consent. Once the patient has been provided the necessary information, the patient has the right to choose what treatments they will receive. They are free to make this decision without pressure from the health care staff. Once they have made this decision, it cannot be undermined unless the patient makes the decision to change treatments. Conversely, if the patient decides to stop the treatment, they may do so, though the doctor should remind the patient about the risks and benefits involved in discontinuing the treatment.

RESPECTFUL CARE

When a patient enters the hospital, they have the right to be treated **respectfully** by those who are providing their care. The patient cannot be discriminated against because of age, gender, race, or religion. They also cannot be denied treatment as a result of the circumstances surrounding their hospitalization. For example, the patient cannot be denied care for injuries acquired during the commission of a crime. While the patient is in the hospital, they have the right to expect care to be provided safely by competent staff. While the patient is in the hospital or extended-care facility, reasonable measures should be taken to accommodate the patient's cultural or religious requests, provided they do not interfere with the care of other patients.

ACCESS TO TELEPHONE AND MAIL

The patient has the right to have regular access to a **telephone** in order to communicate with family members. The patient should be informed as to where the telephone is located and how to use it. The patient should also have an expectation of privacy during his telephone conversations. The patient's conversations should not be monitored or recorded in any way.

The patient has similar rights regarding the **mail**. Patient mail should not be opened without their consent, and any outgoing mail should be sent without being read by members of the health care staff.

CONTINUITY OF CARE

Continuity of care is defined as high-quality health care provided continuously and consistently. Often, continuity of care can be difficult to achieve in a health care setting because of the number of practitioners that can get involved in a patient's case. Continuity of care may break down for a number of reasons, including a doctor's lack of familiarity with a treatment plan or lack of communication among the health care team. In order to maintain continuity of care, there should be frequent conferences between the health care team and the patient to ensure that everyone is in agreement regarding the plan of care.

PATIENT'S RIGHT TO SEE THEIR CHART

If the patient demands to see their chart, the nurse aide should notify the charge nurse. Though it is the patient's **right to see their chart**, most facilities have a policy regarding patient chart review. Such a request is typically forwarded to the medical records department, who will make copies of the patient's chart to provide to the patient. This prevents the patient from potentially altering the information in their chart. Copies of the chart are typically provided within 10 days of the initial request. There may be forms for the patient to fill out prior to receiving copies of the chart, and the charge nurse or someone from the medical records department will provide the forms for the patient.

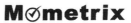

PATIENT'S RIGHTS REGARDING EXPERIMENTAL TREATMENT

The patient has very specific rights when it comes to **experimental treatment**. Like any other procedure, informed consent is required prior to beginning treatment. The patient should be notified of the experimental nature of the treatment, as well as any potential risks and benefits involved in accepting the treatment. The patient should be approached in a manner that is not threatening. If the patient refuses the treatment, they have the right to be informed of other treatments that may be performed in place of the experimental treatment. Care cannot be refused to the patient based upon refusal of an experimental treatment.

PATIENT'S RIGHT OF REFUSAL

If the patient is alert and oriented, they have the **right to refuse** any treatment or procedure. This includes simple procedures, such as turning or a bath. If the patient decides, for example, that they do not want to be turned, they should not be scolded or coerced for this decision. They should be informed of the risks involved in not being turned. If the patient continues to refuse, then the nurse aide should not argue. The charge nurse should be notified so that the proper documentation can be made. If possible, the nurse aide may offer the procedure again at a later time.

PATIENT'S RIGHT TO LEAVE THE HEALTH CARE FACILITY

As long as the patient is alert and oriented, they may choose to **leave the health care facility** at any time. If the patient states a desire to leave, the nurse aide should inform the charge nurse immediately. The charge nurse will talk to the patient and attempt to discover the reason that they want to leave. If the patient cannot be convinced to stay and is considered competent to make that decision, the doctor will be notified of the patient's decision. In many cases, the patient will be asked to sign an AMA form, indicating that they acknowledge that they are leaving Against Medical Advice. It is not the responsibility of the nurse aide to obtain the patient's signature.

PATIENT'S RIGHTS REGARDING MONEY AND VALUABLES

Though it is unwise to bring a large sum of **money or valuables** to a hospital setting, it is sometimes unavoidable. Dentures and hearing aids, for example, are very costly pieces of equipment, but they are also necessary for everyday use. If the patient enters the hospital with money or valuables, they have the right to expect that the hospital will take reasonable steps to protect this property. The patient has the right to maintain their own accounts when they enter a long-term care facility. At no point should a member of the health care facility access the patient's financial accounts. If the patient is unable to take responsibility for their financial matters, a social worker should be contacted to make necessary arrangements.

PROTECTING PATIENT VALUABLES

If the patient comes into the hospital with large sums of money or jewelry, the patient should be encouraged to give it to a family member to take home. If a family member is not present, permission should be obtained from the patient to put the **valuables** in the hospital safe. If the patient consents, security should be called, the items catalogued, and a receipt given to the patient. If the patient is unconscious or comatose, the valuables should be locked up until they are able to give consent. If the patient has a valuable that is required for daily use, such as glasses, hearing aids, or dentures, every effort must be taken to protect these items. The patient should be provided a case marked with his name on it. When the items are not in use, they should be kept close at hand in a place where they are not at risk for breaking or being lost.

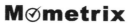

PATIENT'S RIGHT TO IDENTIFICATION OF HEALTH CARE WORKERS

The patient has the right to know the names of the people that are providing their care. On a given day, the patient may encounter a number of people, including doctors, nurses, physical therapists, and nurse aides. A name badge clearly identifies a person as an employee of the health care facility and states the individual's position. It informs the patient of what to expect from the employee. When nurse aides enter the patient's room, they should wear their nametag above the waist in a location that is clearly visible. They should also identify themselves in order to prevent confusion.

RIGHTS OF DYING PATIENTS

A patient's rights should be closely respected at all times, especially when he or she is **dying**. Every effort should be made to place the patient in a private room. When the family is present, the door to the room should be closed; if the door cannot be closed, then the curtain should be pulled shut. Reports regarding the patient should be given where others cannot overhear. Any monitor alarms should be turned off or silenced. Privacy should be respected if the patient needs to be cleaned up and during postmortem care. When transporting the body to the morgue, the morgue cart should be kept covered to protect the patient's identity.

MEDICAL DURABLE POWER OF ATTORNEY

A medical durable power of attorney designates a specific person to make any medically related decisions if the patient should become unable to make the decisions himself. Durable power of attorney would take effect if the patient were to become confused or comatose. The durable power of attorney is typically filed by a lawyer prior to hospitalization. The person who has been made medical power of attorney should make an effort to learn the patient's wishes regarding health care decisions. If the patient becomes hospitalized, the family should present the durable power of attorney paperwork as soon as possible. If the patient's family brings in a copy of the patient's durable power of attorney, the nurse aide should inform the nurse immediately. There can be conflicts regarding power of attorney privileges and patients have the right to change power of attorney, but updated paperwork is required to reflect this change. The patient also must be of sound mind to do so. Any conflicts should be directed to the charge nurse.

ADVANCED DIRECTIVES

Advanced directives detail the patient's wishes regarding end-of-life care. They address whether the patient wants to receive long-term mechanical ventilation, continuous dialysis, or nourishment via a feeding tube. The advanced directives may also address whether the patient wants to be an organ or tissue donor after death. The patient typically sees a lawyer to have his advanced directives prepared prior to hospitalization. Health care providers should be made aware immediately upon hospitalization if the patient has advanced directives. If the patient's family brings in a copy of the patient's advanced directives, the nurse aide should notify the nurse immediately.

DNR ORDER

A Do Not Resuscitate (DNR) order outlines the type of heroic measures that may be undertaken if the patient's heart or breathing were to stop during the course of treatment. The DNR order typically specifies if the patient desires emergent intubation, CPR, or defibrillation. The doctor typically writes a DNR order after an extensive conversation with the patient about his wishes regarding his care. In some cases, the patient may choose to have some of the emergency treatments, but not all of them. It is important for the nurse aide to familiarize oneself with the types of emergency treatment the patient wants. The patient can reverse a DNR at any time. If the patient verbalizes a desire to change their code status, the charge nurse should be notified.

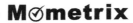

PROTECTING RIGHTS OF PATIENTS WITH DISABILITIES

Every effort should be taken to protect the rights of patients with disabilities. If the patient is hearing or visually impaired, the health care team should tailor its communication techniques to make sure the patient understands what is being said to them. If the patient is confused or mentally challenged, the patient's health care proxy must be kept informed of his or her status and conferred with regarding aspects of care. If the patient does not have a health care proxy and there is no family available, a temporary proxy can be named to act in the patient's best interests until the patient is well enough to do so oneself. If necessary, the health care facility's social work team should be notified to aid in protecting the rights of a patient with disabilities.

PATIENT RESPONSIBILITIES

RESPONSIBILITIES REGARDING THEIR CARE

The health care facility must make every reasonable effort to provide treatment for the patient. However, an optimal level of health cannot be achieved without the assistance of the patient. The patient must actively participate in their care in order for treatment to be successful. Much like the patient's Bill of Rights, the list of **patient responsibilities** should be provided to the patient on admission to the health care facility. These responsibilities include honesty and respect for health care providers, compliance with the treatment plan, meeting financial obligations, not putting others at risk, and responsible decision making. Failure to perform these responsibilities may result in the inability of the health care facility to provide adequate treatment.

MAINTAINING HEALTHY LIFESTYLE

The key to maintaining a **quality lifestyle** is maintaining healthy habits. Healthy habits include a proper diet, exercise, and appropriate lifestyle choices. Though members of the health care team can provide information and encouragement regarding a healthy lifestyle, only the patient can make the necessary changes. It is the responsibility of the health care staff to review the treatment plan and provide education regarding necessary lifestyle changes. However, the treatment is only effective as long as the patient is compliant. If the patient chooses to refuse to follow the treatment plan, they must take responsibility if the plan were to fail.

RESPECT AND HONESTY

It is the patient's right to expect his health care providers to behave in a manner that is polite and respectful; the patient also has a responsibility to behave in a manner that is **respectful toward the health care providers**. Though hospitalization is a stressful time for a patient, it does not excuse disrespectful behavior. Swearing, sexual harassment, and violence are unacceptable behaviors. Acting in such a way makes it difficult for the health care team to provide adequate care. If the patient exhibits behavior that is inappropriate, it should be addressed immediately to make sure it does not interfere with his care.

It is also important for the patient to be **honest** when interacting with the health care staff. The patient should be forthright when answering questions regarding medical and social history, as this information is vital in planning the patient's care. Without all of the necessary information, the planned treatment may be inadequate or may cause harm to the patient.

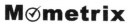

INFORMED DECISION-MAKING

It is the patient's right to determine the type of care she receives. While it is the responsibility of the health care team to provide adequate information to allow the patient to make a decision regarding treatment, it is the patient's responsibility to **make that decision responsibly**. If there is an aspect of the treatment plan that is unclear, the patient should ask questions in order to seek clarification. It is also the patient's responsibility to make decisions regarding treatment based upon the information that has been provided to them, rather than basing decisions on emotions.

ADVANCE DIRECTIVES

In accordance to Federal and state laws, individuals have the right to self-determination in health care, including the right to make decisions about end of life care through **advance directives** such as living wills and the right to assign a surrogate person to make decisions through a durable power of attorney. Patients should routinely be questioned about an advanced directive as they may present at a healthcare provider without the document. Patients who have indicated that they desire a do-not-resuscitate (DNR) order should not receive resuscitative treatments for terminal illness or conditions in which meaningful recovery cannot occur. Patients and families of those with terminal illnesses should be questioned as to whether the patients are Hospice patients. For those with DNR requests or those withdrawing life support, staff should provide the patient palliative rather than curative measures, such as pain control and/or oxygen, and emotional support to the patient and family. Religious traditions and beliefs about death should be treated with respect.

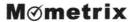

Legal Behavior

REGULATION OF NURSING BY STATES' NURSE PRACTICE ACT

Each state's **nurse practice act** seeks to regulate nursing within the state. It specifies the amount and type of education required to become an RN or LPN/LVN. It defines the nurse's role and responsibilities in healthcare settings. It lists actions that the nurse may take and defines advanced practice education, experience, responsibilities, and limitations. It gives nurses the authorization to perform as required. It also regulates delegation and supervision responsibilities of the nurse. Nurse practice acts are administrated by the state board of nursing, which is responsible for issuing and renewing nurse licenses as well as discipline and censure of nurses. Most state boards of nursing now have a website that provides state-specific information about licensure and nursing rights and responsibilities.

NURSE'S ACCOUNTABILITY FOR NURSING CARE

Nurses are part of an interdisciplinary team responsible for patient outcomes. Nurses have the responsibility for the outcomes of nursing care as a professional group. This responsibility is outlined in each state's nurse practice act, the American Nurses Association (ANA) practice guidelines, and the nurse's job description. Tools, such as the nursing care plan that includes standardized nursing diagnoses, interventions, and expected outcomes, enable the nurse to fulfill this responsibility. Empowerment to act as the patient advocate allows the nurse to point out factors in the patient's individual situation that can be addressed to further improve outcome. Critical thinking during decision-making and detailed documentation are also important. The nurse is held accountable for delegation as well as supervising care by others and evaluation of the outcomes of that care as well. The nurse has personal **accountability** in terms of ethical and moral conduct. Since clinical knowledge is crucial to critical thinking, the nurse must strive to increase knowledge continuously through professional development throughout his or her career.

HIPAA

The Health Insurance Portability and Accountability Act (HIPAA) and state laws govern **who may receive healthcare information** about a person, how permission is to be obtained, how the information may be shared, and patients' rights concerning personal information. HIPAA strives to protect the **privacy** of an individual's healthcare information. Facilities must prevent this information from being accessed by unauthorized personnel. Healthcare information is required to be protected on the **administrative**, **physical**, and **technical** levels. The patient must sign a release form to allow any sharing of patient information. There are stiff penalties for violation of these laws, ranging from $100 for an unintentional violation to $50,000 for a willful violation. Facilities that violate HIPAA may also be subject to corrective actions. Penalties are governed by the Department of Health and Human Services' Office for Civil Right and the state attorneys general.

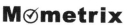

APPLICATION OF HIPAA TO PRACTICE

As an integral member of the health care team, the nurse must always be aware of HIPAA regulations and apply this knowledge to practice. The nurse is responsible for the following efforts to protect and maintain patient privacy:

- The nurse must read and follow facility policies regarding the transfer of patient data.
- Communication between health care personnel about a patient should always be in a private place so that this information is not overheard by those who do not have the right to share the information.
- Access to charts must be restricted to only those health care team members involved in that patient's care.
- Patient care information for unlicensed workers cannot be posted at the bedside, but must be on a care plan or the patient chart in a protected area.
- The nurse must not give information casually to anyone (e.g., visitors or family members) unless it is confirmed that they have the right to have that information.
- Family members must not be relied upon to interpret for the patient; an interpreter must be obtained to protect patient privacy.
- Computers with patient information must have passwords and safeguards to prevent unauthorized access of patient information.
- The nurse should not leave voicemail messages containing protected healthcare information for a patient but should instead ask the patient to call back.

> **Review Video: What is HIPAA?**
> Visit mometrix.com/academy and enter code: 412009

OSHA

The **Occupational Safety and Health Act (OSHA)** seeks to keep workers safe and healthy while on the job. OSHA mandates that employers maintain a safe environment, workers are made fully aware of any hazards, and that access to personal protective gear is made available to workers who come into contact with hazardous materials. By following these regulations, an employer keeps injury and illness of workers to an absolute minimum. This fosters productivity, since workers are not absent due to illness or injury, employee health costs are contained, and the turnover rate is decreased, saving money spent on hiring and training new employees. OSHA is concerned about healthcare employee exposure to radiation, as well as chemical and biological agents, when caring for patients. Information is available to help hospitals and other facilities write plans that comply with best practices to deal with this and other threats to employees. Cleaning procedures, decontamination, and hazardous waste disposal are all covered by OSHA and apply to everyday hospital operation as well as disaster situations.

> **Review Video: What is OSHA (Occupational Safety and Health Administration)**
> Visit mometrix.com/academy and enter code: 913559

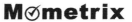

CMS

The **Centers for Medicare and Medicaid (CMS)**, part of the U.S. Department of Health and Human Service department, see to it that healthcare regulations are observed by healthcare facilities that receive federal reimbursement. They reimburse facilities for care given to Medicare, Medicaid, and the state Children's Health Insurance Program (CHIP) recipients. They also monitor adherence to HIPAA regulations concerning healthcare information portability and confidentiality. CMS examines documentation of patient care when deciding to reimburse for care given. CMS has regulations for all types of medical facilities, and these regulations have profoundly impacted nursing practice because nurses must ensure that they comply with regulations related to the quality of patient care and concerns regarding cost-containment. Each facility should provide guidelines to assist nursing staff in meeting the specific documentation requirements of CMS.

OBRA 1987

The **Omnibus Budget Reconciliation Act of 1987 (OBRA 1987)**, also known as the Nursing Home Reform Act, instituted requirements for nursing homes with the purpose of strengthening and protecting patient rights. These requirements are as follows: "a facility must provide each patient with a level of care that enables him or her to attain or maintain the highest practicable physical, mental, and psychosocial wellbeing." OBRA 1987 required that all nursing home patients receive an initial evaluation with yearly follow-ups. Every patient is required to have a comprehensive care plan. Patients were ensured the right to medical care and the right to be informed about and refuse medical treatment. OBRA 1987 requires each state to establish, monitor, and enforce its own licensing requirements in addition to federal standards. Each state is also required to fund, staff, and maintain investigative and Ombudsman units.

OBRA 1990 (PSDA)

The Omnibus Budget Reconciliation Act of 1990 included the amendment called the **Patient Self Determination Act (PSDA)**. The PSDA required healthcare facilities to provide written information about advanced healthcare directives and the right to accept or reject medical or surgical treatments to all patients. Patients who make an advanced directive are leaving instructions about what medical interventions they authorize or refuse if they are incapacitated by illness or injury. They can also nominate another person to make these decisions for them in this situation. The PSDA also protected the right of patients to accept or refuse medical treatments. Healthcare facilities and hospitals are legally required to communicate these rights to all patients, to respect these rights, and to educate staff and personnel about these rights.

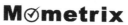

EMTALA

The **Emergency Medical Treatment and Active Labor Act (EMTALA)** is designed to prevent patient "dumping" from emergency departments (ED) and is an issue of concern for risk management that requires staff training for compliance:

- Transfers from the ED may be intrahospital or to another facility.
- Stabilization of the patient with emergency conditions or active labor must be done in the ED prior to transfer, and initial screening must be given prior to inquiring about insurance or ability to pay.
- Stabilization requires treatment for emergency conditions and reasonable belief that, although the emergency condition may not be completely resolved, the patient's condition will not deteriorate during transfer.
- Women in the ED in active labor should deliver both the child and placenta before transfer.
- The receiving department or facility should be capable of treating the patient and dealing with complications that might occur.
- Transfer to another facility is indicated if the patient requires specialized services not available intrahospital, such as to burn centers.

AHRQ

The **Agency for Healthcare Research and Quality (AHRQ)** is part of the U.S. Department of Health and Human Services. This agency is concerned about health care and primarily promotes scientific research into the safety, effectiveness, and quality of healthcare. It encourages evidence-based healthcare that produces the best possible outcome while containing healthcare costs. It makes contracts with institutions to review any published evidence on healthcare in order to produce reports used by other organizations to write guidelines. The agency operates the National Guideline Clearinghouse, which is available online. It is a repository of evidence-based guidelines that address various health conditions and diseases. These guidelines are written by many different health-related professional organizations and are used by primary healthcare providers, nurses, and healthcare facilities to guide patient treatment and care.

STANDARDS OF CARE

Standards of care provide a guideline that explains how a nurse aide is expected to act in a given situation. The state government or the health care facility in which the nurse aide is practicing typically sets these standards. It is the responsibility of the nurse aide to be aware of the appropriate standards of care. If the nurse aide were to fail to act appropriately in a given situation, they could be held responsible for any harm that might come to the patient as a result of them deviating from the expected way to practice.

CIVIL AND CRIMINAL COURT CASES

There are two different types of court cases:

- **Civil court cases** take place between two people, when a wronged individual sues the person who did them wrong. If the accused is found guilty in a civil case, they are typically made to pay fines and restoration to the wronged party.
- In a **criminal court case**, the defendant is accused of committing crimes against society as a whole. If a person is found guilty in a criminal case, they are made to pay fines or serve time in jail.

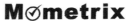

LIABILITY

Liability refers to the responsibility of a person to act within the confines of the law. In the eyes of the law, a person must take responsibility for their own actions. If a nurse aide fails to perform a task to the best of their ability and harm comes to the patient, they can be considered liable. Similarly, if the nurse aide performs a task that falls outside their scope of practice and harm comes to the patient, they are considered liable. In order to maintain safe practice, it is important for a nurse aide to perform tasks exactly as they learned them, without taking shortcuts. The nurse aide should also make an effort to keep their skills and knowledge up to date with current health care trends.

ASSAULT

Assault refers to the threat or attempt to touch or inflict physical harm on another person. The threat could be verbal or physical, such as a threatening gesture or advancing toward a person in a threatening way. Caution must be taken while caring for a patient; if the patient refuses a treatment and the nurse aide attempts to force the patient to receive the treatment, the aide may be liable for assault. It is important to remember that the patient does not have to be harmed in order for the nurse aide to be found liable for assault. It is only necessary to prove that the patient felt threatened in a particular situation.

TORT

A tort is a wrong that is committed in a civil case. There are two types of torts: unintentional and intentional.

- In an **unintentional tort**, a person commits a wrong against another person without intending to cause harm. For example, if a nurse aide forgets to put the side rails back up on the bed and the patient falls and is injured as a result, that could be considered an unintentional tort.
- An **intentional tort** occurs when a person has the intention of causing harm to another person. An example of an intentional tort is if the nurse aide leaves the unit without telling anybody, and the patient becomes injured while they are not being monitored.

NEGLIGENCE

Negligence is the failure to perform care in the manner in which that person was trained. A nurse aide can be charged with negligence if they do not act in a way that is reasonable for a person with their level of training. For example, if the nurse aide leaves a patient unattended in the shower and the patient falls and is injured, the nurse aide could be found negligent. A nurse aide can avoid being accused of negligence by performing procedures exactly as they learned how to do them, without taking shortcuts. If the nurse aide is unsure how to perform a procedure, they should not hesitate to ask for assistance.

BATTERY

Battery refers to the act of touching a person without permission. It could refer to a violent act or an unintended act. A nurse aide might also be accused of battery for performing a procedure on a patient without consent. In order to protect oneself from being accused of battery, a nurse aide should take a moment to explain the procedure to the patient prior to beginning and obtain consent from the patient to perform the procedure. If the patient refuses the procedure, the nurse aide should try to explain the reasons why the procedure is necessary but should not attempt to force the patient to have the procedure performed.

DEFAMATION

When a person makes statements about another person that causes damage to the individual's reputation, they can be accused of defamation.

- **Slander** refers to spoken defamation. For example, if a nurse aide spreads rumors that a patient has HIV, that nurse aide can be accused of slander. A nurse aide can avoid being accused of slander by avoiding saying negative things about other people. By spreading rumors, the nurse aide is acting unprofessionally and is at risk for being accused of defamation.
- **Libel** refers to a written statement that causes injury to another person's reputation. For example, if the nurse aide writes an article that a doctor is practicing without appropriate licensure and that article is untrue, they can be accused of libel.

INVASION OF PRIVACY

The patient has a right to keep details about himself or herself private. **Invasion of privacy** refers to failure to maintain the patient's right to privacy by relaying personal information without the patient's consent. The patient's privacy can be invaded if the nurse aide shares details about the patient's health history with others or by inadvertently leaving sensitive documents where others can easily see them. A nurse aide can avoid being accused of invasion of privacy by only discussing details of the case with those who are directly involved in the care of the patient. If a person who the patient has not identified as one who can receive their information wants details regarding the patient's treatment, the nurse aide should refer them to the charge nurse.

MALPRACTICE

Malpractice is a **type of negligence** that is committed by a professional who needs to maintain a license in order to practice. In a case of malpractice, a professional fails to act according to standards of care within their profession, which results in harm to the patient. Malpractice is more severe than negligence; it takes into account the professional's higher level of training when considering the wrong that was committed by the health care professional. Nurse aides cannot be sued for malpractice, as they are only required to maintain certification. However, they can still be sued for negligence.

FRAUD

Committing **fraud** is deliberately misrepresenting oneself for personal gain. Fraud can be considered a violation of either civil or criminal law. A nurse aide would commit fraud if they claimed to be a nurse or a doctor in the presence of a patient. It is also considered fraud to lie about one's qualifications or certifications on a resume in order to secure a job. A nurse aide can avoid being accused of fraud by clearly identifying oneself when dealing with a patient. They can also avoid being accused of fraud by acting within their scope of practice.

ABANDONMENT

Abandonment occurs when a nurse aide leaves without notifying others or securing another person to provide care in their place. If harm befalls a patient while the nurse aide is absent of their duties, the aide can be accused of abandonment. A nurse aide can avoid being accused of abandonment by asking another nurse aide to cover their patients and informing the charge nurse prior to leaving the unit. They should also make an effort to make sure all of their patients are safe and secure prior to giving report and leaving the unit.

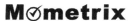

FALSE IMPRISONMENT

False imprisonment refers to confining a person to an area against their will. It is typically used in reference to use of restraints. Restraints are an acceptable tool to be used as a last resort in order to protect both the patient and the safety of others. False imprisonment refers to the use of restraints without an order or in a situation in which it is inappropriate to restrain the patient. A patient could also be falsely imprisoned if they are confined to the health care facility when they wish to leave. If the patient expresses a desire to leave the hospital and is alert and able to make decisions, then the nurse aide should avoid attempting to force the patient to stay. Instead, the aide should notify the charge nurse or the supervisor immediately.

THEFT

Theft is the removal of another person's money or belongings without their knowledge. A nurse aide is guilty of theft if they take a patient's belongings, even if the stolen item is not being used or is not of significant monetary value. Though the health care facility takes steps to avoid hiring people who might steal from patients, the nurse aide should be vigilant as well. The nurse aide should try to avoid theft by not leaving the patient's belongings in plain sight when they are not in use. If the aide sees someone stealing a patient's belongings or acting suspiciously, they should report the behavior to the charge nurse immediately.

LEGAL RAMIFICATIONS OF ABUSE, NEGLECT, AND MISAPPROPRIATION OF PROPERTY

A nurse aide whom is guilty of abuse, neglect, and/or misappropriation of property may be liable to both criminal and civil penalties, depending on the type of act, the result, and the intention. Abuse of a patient (especially if it involved assault and battery or negligence and resulted in injury) and stealing from a patient are criminal offenses for which the nurse aide may be arrested and charged. Non-criminal offenses, such as invasion of privacy, defamation of character, and libel, may result in a civil suit against not only the nurse aide but also those responsible for delegating care, including supervising nurses and the organization. For that reason, if a nurse aide commits or is suspected of non-criminal offenses, the nurse aide is likely to lose employment, even if no civil complaint is filed. If found guilty of a non-criminal act, the nurse aide has to pay a fine and may lose his or her employment and certification.

GRIEVANCE AND DISPUTE RESOLUTION

Grievance and dispute resolution is utilized when one or more parties believe that an agreement (work responsibilities, compensation) has been breached or treatment has been unfair or biased. Each organization should have a procedure in place for reporting grievances/disputes. Procedures usually begin with reporting the problem through the chain of command and/or to the human resources department. In some cases, the dispute may be resolved through supervisorial decision and direction, but with more complex issues, when agreement cannot be reached, or when the proposed agreement is unsatisfactory, the issue may be referred for a further process:

- **Mediation**: A facilitator helps the different parties to the grievance/dispute to discuss the issues and reach a satisfactory resolution. If unsuccessful, further action (arbitration, civil suit) may be needed.
- **Arbitration**: A neutral party listens to both parties to the grievance/dispute and makes a decision, which is usually binding.

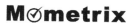

Ethical Behavior

ETHICAL PRINCIPLES

Autonomy is the ethical principle that the individual has the right to make decisions about his or her own care. In the case of children or patients with dementia who cannot make autonomous decisions, parents or family members may serve as the legal decision maker. The nurse must keep the patient and/or family fully informed so that they can exercise their autonomy in informed decision-making.

Justice is the ethical principle that relates to the distribution of the limited resources of healthcare benefits to the members of society. These resources must be distributed fairly. This issue may arise if there is only one bed left and two sick patients. Justice comes into play in deciding which patient should stay and which should be transported or otherwise cared for. The decision should be made according to what is best or most just for the patients and not colored by personal bias.

Beneficence is an ethical principle that involves performing actions that are for the purpose of benefitting another person. In the care of a patient, any procedure or treatment should be done with the ultimate goal of benefitting the patient, and any actions that are not beneficial should be reconsidered. As conditions change, procedures need to be continually reevaluated to determine if they are still of benefit.

Nonmaleficence is an ethical principle that means healthcare workers should provide care in a manner that does not cause direct intentional harm to the patient:

- The actual act must be good or morally neutral.
- The intent must be only for a good effect.
- A bad effect cannot serve as the means to get to a good effect.
- A good effect must have more benefit than a bad effect has harm.

NURSING CODE OF ETHICS

There is more interest in the **ethics** involved in healthcare due to technological advances that have made the prolongation of life, organ transplants, prenatal manipulation, and saving of premature infants possible, sometimes with poor outcomes. Couple these with healthcare's limited resources, and **ethical dilemmas** abound. Ethics is the study of **morality** as the value that controls actions. The American Nurses Association Code of Ethics contains nine statements defining **principles** the nurse can use when faced with moral and ethical problems. Nurses must be knowledgeable about the many ethical issues in healthcare and about the field of ethics in general. The nurse must help a patient to reveal their values and morals to the health care team so that the patient, family, and team can resolve moral issues pertaining to the patient's care. As part of the healthcare team, the nurse has a right to express personal values and moral concerns about medical issues.

BIOETHICS

Bioethics is a branch of ethics that involves making sure that the medical treatment given is the most morally correct choice given the different options that might be available and the differences inherent in the varied levels of treatment. In the health care unit, if the patients, family members, and the staff are in agreement when it comes to values and decision-making, then no ethical dilemma exists; however, when there is a difference in value beliefs between the patients/family members and the staff, there is a bioethical dilemma that must be resolved. Sometimes, discussion and explanation can resolve differences, but at times the institution's ethics committee must be brought in to resolve the conflict. The primary goal of bioethics is to determine the most morally correct action using the set of circumstances given.

ETHICAL DECISION-MAKING MODEL

There are many ethical decision-making models. Some general guidelines to apply in using ethical decision-making models could be the following:

- Gather information about the identified problem
- State reasonable alternatives and solutions to the problem
- Utilize ethical resources (for example, clergy or ethics committees) to help determine the ethically important elements of each solution or alternative
- Suggest and attempt possible solutions
- Choose a solution to the problem

It is important to always consider the **ethical principles** of autonomy, beneficence, nonmaleficence, justice, and fidelity when attempting to facilitate ethical decision-making with family members, caregivers, and the healthcare team.

PROFESSIONAL BOUNDARIES

GIFTS

Over time, patients may develop a bond with nurses they trust and may feel grateful to the nurse for the care provided and want to express thanks, but the nurse must make sure to maintain professional boundaries. Patients often offer **gifts** to nurses to show their appreciation, but some adults, especially those who are weak and ill or have cognitive impairment, may be taken advantage of easily. Patients may offer valuables and may sometimes be easily manipulated into giving large sums of money. Small tokens of appreciation that can be shared with other staff, such as a box of chocolates, are usually acceptable (depending upon the policy of the institution), but almost any other gifts (jewelry, money, clothes) should be declined: "I'm sorry, that's so kind of you, but nurses are not allowed to accept gifts from patients." Declining may relieve the patient of the feeling of obligation.

SEXUAL RELATIONS

When the boundary between the role of the professional nurse and the vulnerability of the patient is breached, a boundary violation occurs. Because the nurse is in the position of authority, the responsibility to maintain the boundary rests with the nurse; however, the line separating them is a continuum and sometimes not easily defined. It is inappropriate for nurses to engage in **sexual relations** with patients, and if the sexual behavior is coerced or the patient is cognitively impaired, it is **illegal**. However, more common violations with adults, particularly elderly patients, include exposing a patient unnecessarily, using sexually demeaning gestures or language (including off-color jokes), harassment, or inappropriate touching. Touching should be used with care, such as touching a hand or shoulder. Hugging may be misconstrued.

ATTENTION

Nursing is a giving profession, but the nurse must temper giving with recognition of professional boundaries. Patients have many needs. As acts of kindness, nurses (especially those involved in home care) often give certain patients extra attention and may offer to do **favors**, such as cooking or shopping. They may become overly invested in the patients' lives. While this may benefit a patient in the short term, it can establish a relationship of increasing **dependency** and **obligation** that does not resolve the long-term needs of the patient. Making referrals to the appropriate agencies or collaborating with family to find ways to provide services is more effective. Becoming

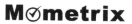

overly invested may be evident by the nurse showing favoritism or spending too much time with the patient while neglecting other duties. On the other end of the spectrum are nurses who are disinterested and fail to provide adequate attention to the patient's detriment. Lack of adequate attention may lead to outright neglect.

COERCION

Power issues are inherent in matters associated with professional boundaries. Physical abuse is both unprofessional and illegal, but behavior can easily border on abusive without the patient being physically injured. Nurses can easily **intimidate** older adults and sick patients into having procedures or treatments they do not want. Regardless of age, patients have the right to choose and the right to refuse treatment. Difficulties arise with cognitive impairment, and in that case, another responsible adult (often the patient's child or spouse) is designated to make decisions, but every effort should be made to gain patient cooperation. Forcing the patient to do something against his or her will borders on abuse and can sometimes degenerate into actual abuse if physical coercion is involved.

PERSONAL INFORMATION

When pre-existing personal or business relationships exist, other nurses should be assigned care of the patient whenever possible, but this may be difficult in small communities. However, the nurse should strive to maintain a professional role separate from the personal role and respect professional boundaries. The nurse must respect and maintain the confidentiality of the patient and family members, but the nurse must also be very careful about **disclosing personal information** about him or herself because this establishes a social relationship that interferes with the professional role of the nurse and the boundary between the patient and the nurse. The nurse and patient should never share secrets. When the nurse divulges personal information, he or she may become vulnerable to the patient, a reversal of roles.

ETHICAL ASSESSMENT

While the terms *ethics* and *morals* are sometimes used interchangeably, ethics is a study of morals and encompasses concepts of right and wrong. When making **ethical assessments,** one must consider not only what people should do but also what they actually do, as these two things are sometimes at odds. Ethical issues can be difficult to assess because of personal bias, which is one of the reasons that sharing concerns with other internal sources and reaching consensus is so valuable. Issues of concern might include options for care, refusal of care, rights to privacy, adequate relief of suffering, and the right to self-determination. Internal sources might include the ethics committee, whose role is to make decisions regarding ethical issues. Risk management can provide guidance related to personal and institutional liability. External agencies might include government agencies, such as the public health department.

ETHICAL ANALYSIS OF A SITUATION

Assessment of the situation is done to reveal the ethical, legal, and professional **conflicts** that are present. Those who are involved are identified, including the patient, family, and healthcare personnel. The decision maker is determined if it is not the patient. Information about the situation is collected to determine medical facts about the disease and condition of the patient, options for treatment, and nursing diagnoses. Any pertinent legal information is included. The patient and family's cultural, religious, and moral values are determined. Possible courses of action are listed and compared in terms of outcomes for the patient using the utilitarian or deontological theory of ethics. Professional codes of ethics are also applied. A decision is made and evaluated as to whether it is the most morally correct action. Ethical arguments for and against the decision are given and responded to by the decision maker.

Member of the Health Care Team

HEALTH CARE TEAM MEMBERS

The health care team is a group of people who provide care for a patient. It includes the patient, the physician, the nurse and other members of the nursing team, and any specialists who may be brought in to participate in caring for the patient.

- The **patient** is the most important member of the health care team; patients consent to any treatments that might be performed and must actively participate in order for treatment to be successful.
- The **physician** diagnoses any diseases or conditions the patient may have and prescribes medications and treatments to treat the patient.
- The **nurse** is responsible for assessing the patient and administering medications.
- The **nurse aide** helps the nurse in providing care to the patient.
- **Specialists** may be consulted to aid in the patient's treatment, such as a physical therapist or a speech therapist.

CERTIFIED NURSE AIDE

ROLE AND REQUIREMENTS FOR CERTIFICATION

A nurse aide is a valuable member of the health care team. The primary **role** of the nurse aide is to assist the nurse in providing care for the patient. The nurse aide's primary responsibility is to see to the patient's basic needs.

The **requirements to become certified** as a nurse aide vary depending upon the state. However, most states require a minimum of 75 hours of training, including classroom instruction and review of basic skills. After the training has been completed, a nurse aide must undergo the state certification exam in order to be qualified to provide care to patients. The test is typically divided into two parts: a written exam and a demonstration of skills.

RENEWING CERTIFICATION

Certification periods for nurse aides are usually for 2 years (the expiration date is on the certificate) after which the certification must be renewed. For **renewal**, the individual must have worked continually or must have met the minimum number of hours required for renewal and must have no substantiated findings of abuse, neglect, or misappropriation of property. If the nurse aide does not meet the minimum work requirements, then the certificate may be declared null or inactive, in which case the individual may be required to reapply and take the certifying examination for renewal. Federal law requires 12 hours continuing education each year for certification renewal, but some states have further requirements, such as additional hours or specific courses that must be taken, so the nurse aide must always check individual state requirements.

CONTINUING EDUCATION REQUIREMENTS

Unless a nurse aide continues to study and learn, their skills will become outdated. The health care facility is required to provide at least 12 hours of **continuing education** every year in order for the nurse aide to keep their skills up to date. Continuing education includes teaching regarding new skills and a review of skills that are already known. It is the responsibility of the nurse aide to provide proof of continuing education in order to maintain certification. If the facility does not offer it, the nurse aide should speak to the supervisor about what can be done to acquire these required continuing education hours.

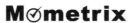

SCOPE OF PRACTICE

Scope of practice is a list of tasks that a nurse aide is allowed to perform as determined by the state certification board. It is the responsibility of the nurse aide to be aware of what tasks they can and cannot perform. Any activity that does not appear on the list falls outside the nurse aide's scope of practice. If the nurse aide is caught performing an activity that is not on the list, they run the risk of losing certification. The nurse aide is liable for any harm that comes to the patient as a result of them performing an activity that is outside their scope of practice.

TASKS NOT PART OF THE NURSE AIDE'S SCOPE OF PRACTICE

There are a number of tasks that **fall outside the nurse aide's scope of practice**. A nurse aide is not allowed to receive orders from a doctor; only a nurse can receive these orders. A nurse aide may not insert or remove devices from a patient's body, such as indwelling catheters, IVs, or rectal tubes. Also, a nurse aide may not perform any sort of sterile procedure. In most cases, a nurse aide may not administer medications. Some states allow a nurse aide to assist the patient in self-administration of medication under specific circumstances. The nurse aide may only assist in medication administration if they receive special training and may only assist in administering certain medications.

RESPONSIBILITIES OF THE NURSE AIDE

The nurse aide's primary **responsibility** is to care for the patient's basic needs. The aide should see to the patient's nutritional needs by distributing the meal trays and feeding the patient if necessary. They should also aid the patient in exercising. Whenever necessary, the nurse aide will aid the patient with elimination and hygiene needs. The nurse aide may be responsible for checking vital signs, answering call lights, and reporting any changes to the charge nurse. There may also be other tasks that will be the nurse aide's responsibility, and these tasks will be detailed by the health care facility.

PRIORITIZATION OF RESPONSIBILITIES

Prioritization of responsibilities involves establishing a sequence for care activities. At the beginning of a shift, the nurse aide should take a few minutes to organize and plan care. Priority should be based on:

1. Duties the **delegating nurse** states have priority should be attended to first.
2. Duties for which a **medical response** may be needed, including vital signs, temperature, and measuring intake and output are usually attended to next.
3. Duties that involve the **patient's health and wellbeing,** such as turning or positioning the patient, ensuring safety, assisting with toileting or exercises, changing adult diapers, and ensuring adequate nutritional and fluid intake.
4. **Routine care duties,** such as mouth care, brushing hair, bathing, and changing linen, are generally the lowest priority, which means they can usually be delayed but not ignored or overlooked.

The nurse aide should also consider the patient's priorities and accommodate them when possible. For example, if a patient is expecting visitors, routine care may be the patient's priority.

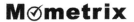

ROLE IN THE PLANNING PROCESS AND IMPLEMENTATION OF CARE PLANS

The nurse aide has an important role in the **planning process** and **implementation of the care plan**. The nurse aide often spends more one-on-one time with patients than licensed personnel, so the aide may have invaluable insights into the patient's progress, abilities, concerns, and emotional status and should share those observations with the nurse and document them so they are part of the permanent record. The nurse aide is often responsible for implementing various aspects of the care plan, such as assisting the patient to sit up or ambulate, monitoring intake and output, promoting comfort, preventing infection, and providing reassurance. In addition to the nursing care plan, which includes problems, interventions, and expected outcomes, the nurse aide should think in terms of individual nurse aide care plans related to the type of care the nurse aide provides when planning care, identifying goals (promote comfort, prevent injury) and interventions appropriate for the patient.

SETTING UP PATIENT'S ROOM

It is important for a patient's **room to be properly set up** prior to their arrival. This ensures the admission process goes as smoothly as possible. When the nurse aide receives word of an admission, they should make sure the room is set up as soon as possible. The bed linens should be turned down. There should be a clean hospital gown in the room in case the patient arrives wearing street clothes or a soiled gown. The room supplies should be stocked. Telemetry equipment and other necessary equipment should be at bedside; this can include a thermometer, sphygmomanometer, or pulse oximetry probe. Miscellaneous equipment, such as oxygen tubing, Foley catheter equipment, a graduated cylinder, and suction equipment should be provided if it is ordered. The nurse aide should also have the packet of admission paperwork at the bedside.

ADDRESSING FAMILY MEMBERS THAT WISH TO PARTICIPATE IN THE PATIENT'S CARE

In some cases, a member of the patient's family may express a desire to **participate in the patient's care**. If a family member makes this request, the nurse aide should notify the charge nurse. Ultimately, the decision about allowing the family member to assist with care depends upon the patient, due to their right to privacy, the patient's condition, and the complexity of the care the family member would like to help with. It may be appropriate for a family member to assist in some cases, such as if the patient were going home soon and would require assistance at home. The nurse should provide instructions to the family member, but the nurse aide should be vigilant while the family member is providing care to ensure that it is being properly done.

REFUSING ASSIGNMENTS
REASONS FOR NURSE AIDES TO REFUSE AN ASSIGNMENT

A nurse aide must have a valid reason to **refuse an assignment**. There are a number of reasons why they might do so. A particular assignment might not be part of an aide's scope of practice. The nurse aide might feel uncomfortable with the assignment as a result of not knowing how to perform a task or may feel it is unethical or illegal. The nurse aide may refuse an assignment if they feel performing the task will cause harm to the patient or may place oneself in danger if they were to perform that task.

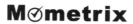

How Nurse Aides Should Refuse an Assignment

A nurse aide should only refuse an assignment if they have a good reason to do so. After the assignments have been made, the nurse aide should talk to the charge nurse privately about their discomfort regarding the assignment. This should be done in a calm manner. The aide should explain their concerns and the reason why they are declining the assignment. The nurse aide and the charge nurse should come to an agreement regarding the assignment. If the nurse aide and the charge nurse are unable to come to an agreement, the nurse aide should clearly state that they are declining the assignment.

Maintaining Good Interpersonal Relationships

Good interpersonal relationships are the key to functional team work. This is necessary in order to provide safe and comprehensive patient care. A nurse aide can maintain good interpersonal relationships in a number of ways.

- Behave with a positive attitude.
- Try to avoid gossiping about coworkers and avoid openly criticizing them.
- Perform any tasks that are assigned promptly and notify the charge nurse if there are any tasks that the aide is unable to perform during the shift.
- Utilize teamwork by regularly offering to provide assistance to others and thanking them for any assistance they provided.

Delegation

Delegation refers to assigning a task to another person. It is within the nurse's scope of practice to assign tasks to the nurse aide and LPN; however, it is not within the nurse aide's scope of practice to assign tasks to others. Though the nurse aide is responsible for performing the task, it is the responsibility of the nurse to make sure that it is done properly and in a timely manner. When assigned a task, the nurse aide should make sure they understand how to perform that task. If they do not know how to do it, the nurse aide should either ask for instructions in order to perform the task safely or decline the assignment.

Professionalism

Topics to Discuss During Job Interview

A **job interview** is a time for an interviewer to meet an applicant, but it is also a good time for an applicant to get to know the interviewer and the place in which they may be working. Before the interview, the nurse aide should think of questions regarding the job description and the facility and write them down. This might include questions about the nurse/patient ratio and the most common types of patients that receive care at the facility. It might also include the number of nurse aides that the facility employs and what the turnover rate is. The aide should avoid asking questions about pay and benefits until after the job offer has been made.

Attire While on Duty

Part of behaving in a professional manner is **dressing appropriately**. Most facilities have a dress code that all employees should follow. The nurse aide should wear scrubs that follow the dress code. The scrubs should be clean and well mended. Though the scrubs need not be pressed, they should be free of wrinkles. Shoes should be clean and comfortable. The nurse aide should also wear minimal jewelry and avoid long necklaces, dangling earrings, and rings. Fragrances and perfumes should also be avoided as some patients have sensitivities to their properties. The nurse aide should keep their nails trimmed and should avoid wearing nail polish or acrylic nails to work.

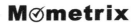

BECOMING ILL PRIOR TO A SCHEDULED SHIFT

A nurse aide should take every precaution to avoid becoming ill. **If the aide becomes ill**, he or she should not report to work, where the illness could possibly be spread to the patient population. Most health care facilities have policies regarding sudden illness, and the nurse aide should make oneself aware of these policies. Most facilities require the nurse aide to provide notification of absence at least two hours prior to the start of the shift. It also may be necessary to provide a doctor's excuse if the illness requires them to miss multiple days of work.

SCHEDULING CONFLICTS

A nurse aide should endeavor to make their supervisor aware of any important events so that the facility might work around those events. However, **scheduling conflicts** do occasionally occur. Most health care facilities have policies regarding scheduling conflicts, and the nurse aide should familiarize oneself with these policies. If a conflict arises, the nurse aide should talk to their colleagues and try to make arrangements to switch workdays in order to accommodate the schedule. If the nurse aide is unable to find someone to switch, they should talk to their supervisor and attempt to make arrangements that can accommodate their schedule. Under no circumstances should the nurse aide not show up for work.

NURSE AIDE REGISTRY

In accordance with federal laws, a **Nurse Aide Registry** is maintained by all 50 states and the District of Columbia, and each has individuals or departments assigned to investigate complaints about nurse aides. Long-term care facilities are required to verify that an individual applying for a position as a nurse aide is certified and has met competency requirements prior to employment. The registry provides information about the individual regarding education, work experience, and any substantiated findings of abuse, neglect, or misappropriation of property (these findings preclude an individual from employment). Copies of disciplinary actions may be available. While state laws may vary somewhat, generally nurse aides must report employment in order to maintain current status. Nurse aides who have been unemployed for extended periods (typically 24 months) may need to take a competency test before certification renewal and listing on the Registry.

EMPLOYER'S RESPONSIBILITIES IN HIRING NURSE AIDES

The employer's responsibilities in hiring a nurse aide include various verification measures that may be carried out by an individual, such as a director of nursing, or by a screening service, such as HireRight:

- **Background check**: Federal law prohibits hiring a nurse aide who has been found guilty of abuse or patient neglect although federal law does not mandate criminal background checks. However, many states require criminal background checks (requiring fingerprinting), and background checks may include the review of sex offender and adult abuse registries. Background checks cannot be used to screen out individuals with health problems or records of receiving Worker's Compensation.
- **References**: All references should be contacted and attempts made to verify that the reference is valid.
- **Registry status**: The Nurse Aide Registry should be checked to verify that the applicant is certified, meets educational requirements, and has no substantiated findings of abuse, neglect, or misappropriation of property.

CNA Practice Test #1

1. When performing a bed bath, what temperature should the water be?

   a. 70-80 degrees Fahrenheit
   b. 105-115 degrees Fahrenheit
   c. 130-140 degrees Fahrenheit
   d. 155-165 degrees Fahrenheit

2. Which of the following tasks is NOT completed during a routine bed bath for a diabetic?

   a. Changing the linens
   b. Inspection and cleansing of skin
   c. Perineal care
   d. Nail care

3. How would you classify a pressure sore that has a pink wound bed, but does not extend through the full thickness of the skin?

   a. Stage I
   b. Stage II
   c. Stage III
   d. Stage IV

4. A patient is scheduled for surgery later in the day. What type of food would you expect on his breakfast tray?

   a. No tray – the patient is NPO
   b. Jell-O and chicken broth
   c. Scrambled eggs
   d. French toast and fruit

5. How can a CNA help prevent the development of pressure sores?

   a. Turning the patient every four hours
   b. Providing a full bed bath three times a day
   c. Doing partial baths every time a patient soils herself
   d. Reducing the amount of fluids the patient drinks to minimize incontinence

6. When is it acceptable for a CNA to wash her hands using an alcohol-based hand sanitizer instead of soap and water?

   a. Before eating
   b. After performing peri care on a patient
   c. After using the bathroom
   d. Between checking on patients

7. A CNA is providing care for a patient on contact precautions. What type of personal protective equipment should she be using?

   a. Respirator
   b. Mask
   c. Gown
   d. All of the above

8. Before entering a patient's room, personal protective equipment (PPE) should be put on in which order?
   a. Gown, mask, gloves
   b. Gown, gloves, mask
   c. Mask, gown, gloves
   d. Mask, gloves, gown

9. When changing linens in an isolation room, which of the following is an appropriate measure to prevent contamination of clean materials?
   a. Placing dirty linens in a plastic bag inside of the patient's room, and then putting the plastic bag into a bag outside of the room that is held open by a second CNA
   b. Shaking out soiled linens to remove solid material before washing
   c. Piling soiled linens outside of the dirty utility room to avoid mixing them with non-contaminated linens
   d. Moving the soiled linens to the dirty utility room before hand washing

10. Which of the following items requires cleaning with a disinfectant prior to use?
    a. Stethoscope
    b. Scalpel
    c. Thermometer
    d. Blood pressure cuff

11. What is the proper term for an infection that is transmitted during a medical procedure?
    a. Droplet
    b. Iatrogenic
    c. Direct oral contact
    d. Fecal-oral transmission

12. For a patient on fall precautions, what is the minimum number of side rails that should be raised while the patient is in bed?
    a. 1
    b. 2
    c. 3
    d. 4

13. Before transferring a patient from the bed to a wheelchair, what is the very first thing the CNA should do?
    a. Place her arms under the patient's axilla and assist her to a standing position.
    b. Assist the patient to a sitting position.
    c. Allow the patient to dangle her legs for a few minutes before standing.
    d. Ensure the wheels on both the wheelchair and the bed are locked.

14. What type of assistance would be required for an elderly woman who fell recently, but is still able to ambulate?
    a. Stand by assistance
    b. Minimum assistance
    c. Contact guard assistance
    d. Maximum assistance

15. Which technique is MOST appropriate for a patient with both poor upper body and lower body strength?

    a.   Four-point technique
    b.   Three-point technique
    c.   Swing-to method
    d.   Swing-through method

16. A CNA encounters a small fire in a patient's room. The room is empty. What is her first priority?

    a.   Rescue patients in the neighboring rooms
    b.   Activate the fire alarm
    c.   Close all fire doors
    d.   Grab a fire extinguisher and attempt to extinguish the fire

17. Which of the following procedures is NOT appropriate for a patient who has been ordered to be placed in restraints?

    a.   Offer toileting and water every one to two hours
    b.   Check the patient at least every 30 minutes to ensure there is proper circulation where the restraints are applied
    c.   Tie the restraints directly to the bed frame
    d.   Tie the restraints directly to the side rails

18. How should a CNA clean an indwelling catheter?

    a.   By using a gentle back and forth motion
    b.   By using a circular motion towards the body
    c.   By using a circular motion away from the body
    d.   By using an up and down motion

19. Before taking a meal tray into a patient's room, what should a CNA do?

    a.   Record the amount of food/liquids on the intake/output form
    b.   Assess a patient's ability to swallow properly
    c.   Put on gloves
    d.   Ensure that the correct food is on the tray

20. If a CNA notices that a patient appears to be having difficulty swallowing, what should she do?

    a.   Notify the nurse immediately
    b.   Mash up the food and continue feeding the patient
    c.   Give the patient smaller amounts of food with each bite
    d.   Nothing; the doctor checked the patient's swallowing already

21. How often should anti-embolism stockings be removed?

    a.   Every 4 hours
    b.   Every 8 hours
    c.   Every 12 hours
    d.   Every 24 hours

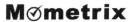

22. There is a note on a patient's chart that she should be placed in the Sim's position. How should the patient be positioned?

    a. Lying on the stomach with the head turned to the side

    b. On her back with the head of the bed raised to a 90-degree angle

    c. On her back with the head of the bed raised to a 45-degree angle

    d. On her left side with the top leg flexed and supported by a pillow

23. What is the first step for a CNA who is about to put on sterile gloves?

    a. Use the dominant hand to grasp the glove at the cuff and slide it on to the non-dominant hand.

    b. Use the non-dominant hand to grasp the glove under the cuff and slide it on to the dominant hand.

    c. Wash and dry hands thoroughly.

    d. Put on gloves to open the packaging.

24. Which of the following is a measurement of the pressure in a patient's heart during contraction?

    a. Systolic blood pressure

    b. Diastolic blood pressure

    c. Apical pulse

    d. Pulse oximetry

25. Which of the following abnormal vital signs should be immediately reported to the nurse?

    a. Oral temperature of 99.2 degrees

    b. Respiratory rate of 5

    c. Blood pressure of 126/72

    d. Pulse rate of 59

26. Which fluids should be included in the measurement of a patient's intake?

    a. 8 oz. of milk

    b. 250 mL of intravenous fluid

    c. 6 oz. of Jell-O

    d. All of the above

27. What is the first thing a CNA should do when measuring a patient's height and weight?

    a. Wash her hands

    b. Verify the patient's identity by inspecting her armband

    c. Allow the patient's legs to dangle for a few moments before allowing her to stand up

    d. Assist the patient with ambulation to the scale

28. Which of the following is an example of subjective data?

    a. The patient has a pulse rate of 88 bpm.

    b. The patient states that she has a pain level of 8.

    c. The CNA notes that the patient has flushed cheeks.

    d. The CNA notes that the patient has cloudy urine.

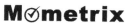

29. While completing her documentation, a CNA notices that she made a mistake while writing in a patient's blood pressure. How should she correct the notation?
  a. Use correction fluid to cover the mistake
  b. Scribble out the incorrect number and write the correct number next to it
  c. Draw a single line through the incorrect notation, and write "error," along with her initials. The correct number should be written next to it
  d. Erase the incorrect notation; documentation is always completed using a pencil

30. A patient with which of the following conditions is MOST at risk for dehydration?
  a. Diarrhea
  b. Liver disease
  c. Heart disease
  d. Pneumonia

31. When caring for a patient with diarrhea, which of the following should be recorded in the patient's chart?
  a. Odor of the stool
  b. Types and amounts of fluids the patient is drinking
  c. Number of stools
  d. All of the above

32. How often should a patient who is lying on an egg crate or an inflatable mattress be turned?
  a. Never – patients shouldn't be turned when they are lying on inflatable mattresses.
  b. Every 12 hours
  c. Every 6 hours
  d. Every 2 hours

33. Which of the following is NOT an intervention a CNA can use to manage edema?
  a. Elevate the affected extremity
  b. Use ice or a cold pack to reduce swelling
  c. Massage the affected extremity using lotion
  d. Encourage activity or use range of motion exercises

34. A patient with a shuffling gait, difficulty swallowing and speaking, and short-term memory loss MOST likely has which of the following?
  a. Alzheimer's disease
  b. Dementia
  c. Parkinson's disease
  d. Sundowner's syndrome

35. A CNA is caring for a patient with Sundowner's syndrome. Which of the following symptoms should he be especially aware of?
  a. Worsening confusion at night
  b. Risk for falls
  c. Aggression
  d. Difficulty swallowing

36. What is one technique a CNA can use to help a patient with aphasia?

    a. Providing a time limit for the patient to respond
    b. Speaking for the patient
    c. Using a picture or letter board
    d. Giving the patient a pen

37. A CNA is caring for a patient who is becoming agitated. How should she speak to the patient?

    a. In an assertive and confident manner
    b. Not at all; the patient's family members or other staff should interact with the patient
    c. She should not acknowledge the inappropriate behavior and carry on as normal
    d. Calmly and clearly, while attempting to determine why the patient is agitated

38. Hospice care is appropriate for which of the following?

    a. Patients who are expected to live less than three months
    b. Patients who are expected to live less than six months
    c. Patients who are actively dying
    d. Patients who have been diagnosed with a terminal disease, regardless of their clinical condition

39. Which of the following answer choices correctly lists the five stages of grief in order of their expected occurrence?

    a. Denial, anger, bargaining, depression, acceptance
    b. Anger, denial, depression, bargaining, acceptance
    c. Depression, denial, anger, bargaining, acceptance
    d. Bargaining, denial, anger, depression, acceptance

40. Unless otherwise ordered, how often should a CNA record the vital signs of a patient who is actively dying? The patient has a signed DNR order in place.

    a. Every 5 minutes
    b. Every 15 minutes
    c. Every hour
    d. Never

41. While you are caring for a Buddhist patient, he mentions an upcoming fast day when he can only eat at predetermined times during the day. What is an appropriate response?

    a. Acknowledge his beliefs but explain that you can't make any changes to the facility's dining times
    b. Suggest that his family bring some food from home
    c. Speak with him to determine what his needs will be that day and coordinate with the dining and food team
    d. Apologize for not being able to help him that day

42. When caring for a Jewish patient who observes the Kosher laws, the CNA notices his dinner plate has a dish with pork in it. What should the CNA do?

    a. Bring him the food tray and see if he requests a change
    b. Call the dining/food department to order a new tray, and explain the delay to the patient
    c. Remove the pork from his plate and serve him the tray
    d. Switch trays with another patient

43. What needs are found on the bottom level (most basic) of Maslow's pyramid?
   a. Physiological
   b. Safety/security
   c. Love and belonging
   d. Self-esteem

44. A CNA needs to speak with a patient about the quality and amount of stool he passed that day. How can the CNA help the patient feel more comfortable about disclosing the needed information?
   a. Ask the patient in his room when visitors are present
   b. Ask the patient in the privacy of his room in a quiet tone
   c. Ask the patient in an indirect way and hope the patient understands what the CNA is trying to ask
   d. Ask the patient closed-ended questions

45. A patient states that she is depressed. Which of the following responses by the CNA involves the use of reflection?
   a. I'm sorry that you're feeling depressed.
   b. Why are you feeling depressed? Your recovery is moving along well.
   c. Do you want to speak with someone about this?
   d. You feel depressed?

46. A CNA is stocking shelves outside a patient's room when the call bell rings. The CNA is not responsible for the patient's care that day. How should the CNA respond?
   a. Ignoring the call bell until the patient's assigned CNA responds
   b. Getting the assigned CNA to check on the patient
   c. Checking on the patient right away to see what she needs
   d. Checking on the patient after stocking the shelves

47. A patient has rung the call bell for the sixth time during the first two hours of a CNA's shift. How should she respond?
   a. Ignore the bell
   b. Call the nurse manager
   c. Remove the bell from the patient's reach
   d. Reassure the patient she will be checked on frequently

48. A CNA has been assigned to care for a ventilated patient, which she has never done before. How should she handle the situation?
   a. Notify the nurse manager that she is not sure how to care for the patient, and request additional instructions or training materials
   b. Do the best she can while caring for the patient
   c. Speak with the other CNAs to find out what additional care is needed for the patient
   d. Request to switch patients with another CNA

49. A CNA has to ask a sensitive question to a patient who doesn't speak English. How should she ask the question?
   a. Using the patient's family to translate
   b. Calling the hospital's official translation service
   c. Gesturing to the patient in the hope she will understand
   d. Looking up relevant words on the Internet before speaking with the patient

50. A patient's family asks how he is doing after his scheduled MRI. How should the CNA respond?
   a. He had an MRI today?
   b. His MRI results are back. Everything is normal.
   c. He seems to be in good spirits. Let me see if he's ready to visit with you and I'll find his nurse to talk to you about the results.
   d. Good. He should be ready to go home soon.

51. HIPAA guarantees a patient's right to which of the following?
   a. Confidentiality
   b. Informed consent
   c. See their chart
   d. Continuity of care

52. A patient has a few questions about the consent forms she signed for a scheduled invasive procedure. How should the CNA respond?
   a. Answer the questions to the best of her ability
   b. Tell the patient that she will ask the nurse to contact the doctor
   c. Tell the patient that she will have plenty of time to ask the doctor before the procedure
   d. Remind the patient that she signed the consent and that the procedure has already been scheduled

53. A family member gives a copy of a patient's advanced directives to a CNA. The patient is scheduled for a minor procedure the next day. Which of the following is an appropriate response?
   a. Tell them to hold onto the copies until and unless they are needed
   b. Tell the family that they are not necessary because the patient is having a minor surgical procedure
   c. Put the copy in the chart
   d. Immediately notify the nurse that the family has advanced directives for the patient

54. A patient is refusing to be turned and it has been several hours since he was last turned. The patient is alert and oriented. How should the CNA respond?
   a. Turn him anyway; he needs it to prevent skin breakdown
   b. Inform him that she will tell the doctor he is refusing care so he can go home
   c. Inform him of the associated risks, and then respect his decision if he still does not want to be turned
   d. Tell him whatever is necessary to obtain his consent to be turned

55. Which of the following would NOT be included in a list of patient responsibilities?
   a. Honesty
   b. Polite and respectful behavior
   c. Maintain all personal property
   d. Compliance with treatment plan

56. A nurse asks a CNA to give Tylenol to a patient who has a headache. The nurse is very busy with another critical patient. What should the CNA do?
   a. Administer the Tylenol; the nurse did the assessment and delegated this task to her
   b. Refuse to give the patient any medication – it is not within her scope of practice
   c. Find the Tylenol and repeat the order – including the patient's name, room number, and instructions – back to the nurse to confirm her directions
   d. Ask another nurse to give the medication

57. While in an elevator, another CNA asks you about the MRI results for the patient in room 307. The CNA cared for the patient while on another unit. What is an appropriate response?
   a. Refuse to answer the question; the CNA is no longer an active member of the patient's health care team
   b. Answer the question fully and honestly
   c. Answer the question without using any identifying information so the others in the elevator won't know who you are talking about
   d. Wait until the other people exit the elevator to answer the question

58. A patient who was injured while committing a criminal act has a right to treatment under which of the following patient rights?
   a. Right to freedom of choice
   b. Right to respectful care
   c. Right to continuity of care
   d. Right of refusal

59. A patient demands to see his medical chart. What should the CNA do?
   a. Give the patient his chart and leave the room to give him privacy
   b. Give the patient the chart and stay in the room to ensure he doesn't make any changes
   c. Make photocopies of the chart and give them to the patient
   d. Inform him that he will need to notify the medical records department to make arrangements

60. For what reason would a doctor write a DNR order?
   a. To prevent any care from being provided to a patient.
   b. To explain the care the doctor feels would most benefit a patient.
   c. To explain what type of emergency care a patient wishes to have.
   d. To discharge a patient into hospice care.

61. If a patient refuses a treatment and the CNA attempts to perform it anyway, what could the CNA be charged with?
   a. Assault
   b. Battery
   c. Either A or B
   d. Neither A nor B

117

62. A CNA who forgets to lock the wheels on a wheelchair (which results in a subsequent fall) could be charged with which of the following?

    a. Assault
    b. Battery
    c. Malpractice
    d. Negligence

63. If a CNA observes the nursing supervisor acting in a negligent way, what should she do?

    a. Speak with the doctor in charge of the patient
    b. Follow the institution's chain of command to determine who to report the behavior to
    c. Go to the institution's president of nursing to report the behavior
    d. Confront the nursing supervisor directly

64. If a CNA begins to suspect that a patient is being abused by a family member, what should she do?

    a. Report it to the charge nurse
    b. Report it to the police
    c. Ignore it because the nurse and doctor probably suspect it too
    d. Confront the suspected abuser

65. Who is the most important member of the health care team?

    a. The nurse
    b. The patient
    c. The physician
    d. The CNA

66. What is the minimum number of hours of continuing education that a CNA should complete each year?

    a. 6
    b. 12
    c. 20
    d. 50

67. What is the BEST way for a CNA to assist during a code?

    a. Administer emergency medications according to the physician's instructions
    b. Document the events
    c. Speak with the family and answer their questions about what is happening
    d. Retrieve emergency equipment, including the code cart or intubation box, and carry out other assigned tasks that fall within a CNA's scope of practice

68. A patient's daughter is requesting to perform morning care for her mother. The patient is okay with the request, and it has been cleared with the charge nurse. What should the CNA do?

    a. Refuse to let the daughter assist
    b. Allow her to perform the morning care and leave the room to provide privacy
    c. Allow her to assist with morning care, but stay in the room to ensure it is being done correctly
    d. Request that the nurse supervise the patient's daughter

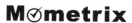

69. When the CNA is informed of an admission, what is her responsibility?

a. Prepare the room, including the linens, gowns, and other necessary equipment
b. Complete the admissions interview
c. Make sure the patient's medications have been received from the pharmacy and are correct
d. Coordinate the patient's care with the rest of the treatment team

70. Which of the following is NOT a reason for a CNA to refuse an assignment?

a. The CNA feels the task is unethical.
b. Performing the task would cause harm to the CNA.
c. The CNA had a serious disagreement with the patient's family the day before.
d. The assignment is outside the CNA's scope of practice.

Answer Key and Explanations for Test #1

1. B: Water for a bed bath should be heated up to approximately 105-115 degrees Fahrenheit. Any cooler and the water will cool off too much before the end of the bath, chilling the patient. Any warmer and the water will be too hot, and could potentially burn the patient. Filling the basin should be the last thing you do; gather all other supplies first to minimize the cooling of the water. If you don't have a thermometer to measure the water temperature, make sure it is comfortably warm against your elbow or inner arm.

2. D: You should check with your institution's policies on nail care, but generally speaking, a CNA should not provide nail care to a diabetic patient. Diabetics have impaired circulation to their extremities, which can delay healing and even cause severe damage if the skin is injured. For that reason, only a physician, podiatrist, or other specially trained clinician should perform nail care on a diabetic. Performing perineal care, changing the linens, and inspecting the skin should be done during every full bed bath, usually as part of morning care.

3. B: A stage I pressure sore would appear as a reddened area that does not blanch (turn white) when pressed. A stage II pressure sore involves a partial breakdown of the upper layer of skin, but does not extend all the way through the skin. A stage II pressure ulcer may look like a blister. Stage III and stage IV ulcers extend all the way through the skin. You may see the underlying subcutaneous fat in a stage III ulcer, whereas a stage IV may proceed all the way down to the muscles, tendons, or bones. Make sure to report any skin redness to the nurse so that the skin can be thoroughly assessed.

4. A: A patient who is about to undergo surgery or another procedure requiring an anesthetic should be NPO for a minimum of eight hours before the procedure. If the patient receives a tray, you should double check with the nurse before serving the patient his breakfast. If a procedure is scheduled for later in the day, the anesthesiologist may be okay with the patient eating breakfast.

5. C: A patient who is bedbound or spends a majority of the day lying or sitting down is at risk for developing pressure sores. Preventing pressure sores requires multiple interventions, including: turning the patient every two hours, doing a full bed bath once a day and partial bed baths throughout the day as necessary if the patient is incontinent (partial baths should be done whenever a patient soils himself), increasing the protein content of food, and making sure the patient is hydrated. It is not appropriate to do a full bed bath twice a day. Withholding fluids to prevent incontinence is also inappropriate.

6. D: Alcohol-based sanitizers are a great tool to avoid the comparatively time-consuming process of hand washing, and are appropriate in certain situations. The CNA should wash her hands with soap and water before eating, after using the bathroom, after performing a procedure that involves contact with bodily fluids (such as peri care), and when her hands are visibly soiled. She should also wash her hands periodically throughout the day to remove the buildup of alcohol on the hands. It is perfectly acceptable to use an alcohol-based sanitizer between checking on patients, especially if the CNA is not performing care.

7. C: If a patient is on contact precautions the caretaker must wear a gown and gloves. Using a mask or respirator is not necessary unless the patient is on droplet or airborne precautions.

8. A: When entering the room of a patient on isolation precautions, the CNA should put on the gown first, with the opening in the back. After tying the gown closed at the neck and around the waist, the

120

mask should be put on next. Lastly, the CNA should put on her gloves, ensuring that the cuff of the gloves is covering the cuff of the gown. When leaving the room, the PPE should be removed in the reverse order: gloves, mask, and gown.

9. A: Anything in the patient's room is considered "contaminated," so when you place the soiled linens into the plastic linen bag, that bag is considered contaminated. The CNA should ask a colleague to hold a second bag open at the doorway and place the contaminated linen bag in it. The second CNA can then put the bag on the floor outside of the room until the first CNA is ready to wash her hands and bring it to the dirty utility room. The soiled linens should never be shaken out because of the risk of contaminating other nearby items.

10. C: Items that require cleaning with a disinfectant are ones that come into contact with a patient's mucus membranes but don't puncture the skin. Thermometers and respiratory equipment are good examples of items that should be disinfected but don't require sterilization. Items such as scalpels that penetrate the skin should be sterilized between patients because of the high risk of contamination. Items such as stethoscopes and blood pressure cuffs that just touch the skin can be cleaned with a mild detergent between uses.

11. B: An infection that is transmitted during a medical procedure is called iatrogenic. Droplet transmission is when bacteria or viruses are released in droplets when a person sneezes or coughs. Direct oral contact is transmission between people when there is direct oral contact, such as kissing or sharing a drinking cup. Fecal-oral contamination is exactly what it sounds like: fecal material contaminates food, usually through poor hand washing or poor food preparation techniques.

12. B: A minimum of two bed rails should be raised when the patient is in bed. Raising four side rails is considered a restraint, and should not be done unless directly ordered by the physician. One raised bed rail leaves an entire side of the bed without any boundaries.

13. D: The very first thing that should be done before transferring a patient is to make sure that the wheels on both the wheelchair and the bed are locked. This prevents falls by preventing movement of the bed or wheelchair as the patient is being transferred. Once the CNA has verified that the wheels are locked, she can help the patient to sit up and allow her to dangle her legs for a few moments. Then, she can help the patient stand up and slide into the wheelchair.

14. C: An elderly woman who has fallen previously is at risk for falling again. However, she is still ambulatory, so the CNA should be within an arm's reach in case the patient becomes unsteady or falls again. This is known as contact guard assistance. Stand by assistance and maximum assistance are inappropriate because they provide too little and too much support, respectively.

15. A: Four-point technique is a great method of crutch walking for patients who have poor upper and lower body strength because it balances out the patient's weight on both arms and the alternating legs. Three-point, swing-to, and swing-through methods are all great for a patient who has good upper body strength because these gaits depend primarily on the arms to keep the patient upright.

16. B: This question can be answered using the acronym R.A.C.E. (rescue, activate alarm, confine the fire, evacuate/extinguish). The CNA should first rescue patients in imminent danger. Because the room is empty, her first priority should be to pull the fire alarm. If the fire is small and contained, she could try to extinguish the fire herself with a fire extinguisher using the P.A.S.S. method (pull the pin, aim at the base of the fire, and sweep side to side). If not, she should start closing fire doors and rescuing patients in neighboring rooms if necessary.

17. D: Whenever a patient is placed in restraints, the CNA should make sure there is an up-to-date order from the physician (within the last 24 hours). The patient should be offered the opportunity to use the bathroom or have a glass of water or food at least every one to two hours. The restraints should be checked at least every thirty minutes to make sure they are not too tight or cutting off circulation to the patient's limbs. The ties should be quick-release knots and the restraints should be tied directly to the bed frame. Restraints should never be tied to the side rails in case they inadvertently fall, which could cause injury to the patient.

18. C: A patient with an indwelling catheter has a higher risk of contracting a urinary tract infection, and so catheter and perineal care is very important. The catheter should be assessed and cleaned frequently. After putting on gloves and explaining what you are going to do, you should use warm water to gently clean the urethra and, using a circular motion away from the body, the catheter. The CNA should never clean upwards or use a back and forth motion because of the potential to introduce bacteria into the urethra. Make sure to dry the catheter and patient, check to make sure there are no kinks in the tubing, and then hang the bag from the bed frame.

19. D: Before taking a meal tray into a patient's room, the CNA should ensure that the tray is labeled with the correct name, room number, and diet. Once she has delivered all of the trays, the CNA can go back and assist patients who need help eating. Ability to swallow should be assessed each time a patient is eating. The CNA should always be alert for signs that the patient isn't swallowing properly. As she is collecting the used food trays, the CNA should document the intake for each patient. This is the best time to see what each patient actually ate.

20. A: Because of the serious risk of aspiration and its complications, the CNA should never continue feeding food to a patient with a suspected swallowing issue. She should immediately stop feeding the patient and notify the nurse. The nurse can inform the doctor and arrange for a swallowing study if necessary, or even change the patient's diet to include soft foods or purées only.

21. B: Anti-embolism stockings should be removed once every eight hours to ensure proper circulation and let the skin breathe. When removing the stockings, the CNA should assess the skin to make sure there are no rashes, skin breakdown, or other concerns. She should also check on the patient's toes to assess blood flow while the stockings are on. If the patient complains of numbness, tingling, or discomfort when wearing the stockings, it should be brought to the nurse's attention immediately.

22. D: Sim's position is when a patient is lying on her side with the top leg flexed towards the chest. Choice A, on her stomach, is called the prone position. Choice B, with the head of the bed raised to a 90-degree angle, is called the High Fowler's position. Choice C, on her back with the head of the bed raised to 45 degrees, is called the Semi-Fowler's position.

23. C: When putting on sterile gloves, the CNA should first wash and dry her hands thoroughly. Then, she should open the packaging, taking care not to touch anything inside. Next, she should pick up the glove for the dominant hand at the cuff using her non-dominant hand and slide it onto the dominant hand. Finally, using the gloved hand, she should pick up the second glove beneath the cuff and slide it onto the non-dominant hand. Once both gloves are on, she can then make adjustments to the fit, taking care to avoid touching anything unsterile.

24. A: Systolic blood pressure, or the top number of the patient's blood pressure, looks at the pressure in the patient's heart during contraction. Diastolic blood pressure, or the lower number, looks at the pressure in the heart during rest. The pulse measures the number of cardiac contractions per minute. Pulse oximetry measures the amount of oxygen in the blood.

25. B: Choices A and D are slightly abnormal and should be reported to the nurse, although it is not necessary to do this immediately. A blood pressure of 126/72 is technically considered abnormal, but can probably be largely attributed to the stress of being in the hospital. It is nothing to be overly concerned about. A respiratory rate of five breaths per minute is very slow, and can indicate impending respiratory failure. The CNA should notify the nurse immediately.

26. D: All of the choices are liquids or melt at room temperature (Jell-O), and should be included in the measurement of a patient's intake. The CNA should also measure the amount of tube feeding (including what is used to flush the tube) and other IV medications or fluids. Total intake should be in mLs and recorded every 24 hours.

27. A: Whenever a CNA enters a patient's room to initiate care or perform a task, she should wash her hands, introduce herself to the patient, and explain what she is going to do. Next, she should identify the patient using the patient's armband and two identifiers. Finally, she can perform the task she came in to do, which in this case is measuring the patient's height and weight.

28. B: Subjective data is anything the patient notes or feels, such as her pain level. Objective data is information that can be measured (such as vital signs) or observed by another person (such as the patient having cloudy urine or flushed cheeks).

29. C: Making documentation errors is common. However, the CNA must understand how to deal with these errors. She should never use correction fluid or scribble out the error so it is illegible. A pencil should never be used for documentation. When an error is made, simply draw a single line through the mistake and place the correction, the word "error," and your initials next to it.

30. A: A patient with diarrhea is at a high risk for dehydration, so all complaints from the patient and direct observations of diarrhea should be reported to the nurse. Signs of dehydration include dry mucus membranes, weakness, and thirst. The CNA may also observe dark urine or sunken eyes. As long as it's not contraindicated, the CNA should encourage the patient to drink extra water to help replace the lost fluids.

31. D: When caring for a patient with diarrhea, it is important to note all of the information in the answer choices in the patient's chart, as it can be vitally important to the care and treatment plan for the patient. Additionally, the doctor will need the information to gauge the severity of the diarrhea and dehydration. The CNA should also note how much fluid is passed with each stool and how often the patient is having episodes of diarrhea.

32. D: Unless the patient is on a special bed that is designed to be used without turning, the patient should always be turned every two hours. Simply adding an egg crate or inflatable mattress to the existing bed is not enough to eliminate or reduce the need to turn the patient. An egg crate can help reduce the pressure on the patient's skin and bony prominences, but the patient should still be turned every two hours.

33. B: True edema is usually a result of poor circulation, so using an ice or cold pack would be of little use in managing it. Useful interventions help stimulate blood flow and blood return. Elevating the extremity will help promote lymphatic drainage and venous return to minimize edema. Movement through ambulation, massage, or range of motion exercises are also great ways to treat and minimize edema.

34. C: All of these symptoms are signs of Parkinson's disease. Alzheimer's disease, dementia, and Sundowner's syndrome all produce similar symptoms, which include confusion, agitation, and wandering. A shuffling gait, though, is the hallmark symptom of Parkinson's disease. A patient with

Parkinson's needs special help with ambulation because their gait is so unsteady, and with eating because they frequently have difficulty swallowing their food.

35. A: Patients with Sundowner's syndrome typically have worsening confusion at night. They may become agitated and wander off the unit. During the day, patients with Sundowner's typically aren't as confused. Possible interventions include checking on and reorienting the patient frequently, and preventing day time sleep so that it is easier for the patient to sleep at night. A patient with Sundowner's may also be at risk for falls or aggression or have difficulty swallowing, but these symptoms are secondary to the confusion they experience at night.

36. C: Aphasia is an acquired inability to understand language and express oneself through speech. Patients with aphasia have different levels of ability, and should be approached with patience. Setting a time limit and speaking for the patient are not productive or helpful in terms of helping the patient relearn these skills. A pen and paper may be helpful in some situations, but many patients aren't able to read or write as a result of their aphasia. A picture or letter board is a universal method of communication, and offers an easy way to communicate because it is so simple to use.

37. D: Patients may become agitated for any number of reasons. They might be in pain or be uncomfortable. They could be hungry, thirsty, have to go to the bathroom, or even be bored or scared. Understanding what is causing someone's agitation is the best way to relieve it. The CNA should continue to interact with the patient in a calm, clear, and professional manner. She may need to set boundaries as necessary, especially if the behavior persists.

38. B: Hospice care is appropriate for patients who are expected to live less than six months. Patients who are transferred into hospice care typically sign a DNR order and are treated using pain relief measures.

39. A: The first stage of grief is denial that the event happened or is going to happen. Following that is anger at the situation or people involved. Next is bargaining, in which the sufferer bargains with God (I'll do...... if you make this go away). Depression follows as the person starts to deal with their grief. Finally, the patient begins to accept what has happened and can start to move forward. It's important to keep in mind that not everyone goes through the same steps in a linear and straightforward manner. It's not uncommon for someone to progress through one stage quickly and then get held up at a subsequent stage or even regress back to a prior stage.

40. D: Generally speaking, the CNA should never record the vital signs of a patient with a DNR order in place who is actively dying. The clinical staff, including the CNA, should do everything in their power to make the patient and their family comfortable. The family may want the extra time with their loved one without being interrupted. Additionally, the act of having their vital signs taken may cause pain or discomfort for the patient, both of which should be avoided if possible. If, however, the physician has ordered otherwise, the CNA should defer to the wishes of the physician and nurse.

41. C: A patient's religion plays a huge role in how well a patient is able to heal and cope with their disease. The CNA should advocate for her patient and arrange for meals to be sent up at the designated times. She could also coordinate with the nurse and other staff members to ensure continuity. Having his family bring food from home may be one possibility, but the CNA should first try to make arrangements with the dining department.

42. B: Kosher dietary laws are strict guidelines that people who belong to the Jewish faith must follow. The CNA should be sensitive to that and arrange for another tray to be sent up from the dining department. It is not appropriate to simply remove the pork from the patient's tray or wait until the patient requests a change. The CNA should not switch his tray with another patient's. Each tray is specially prepared based on patients' nutritional needs and allergies.

43. A: Physiological needs must be met first, and are therefore at the bottom of the pyramid. These needs include food, water, sex, and oxygen. The next level is the need for safety and security. This isn't restricted to just physical security, but also the safety of one's family, morals, finances, employment, and property. Love and belonging (usually to a group such as a family or friends) is the next level. The final two levels are self-esteem (encompassing self-confidence and achievement) followed by self-actualization, which includes creativity, spontaneity, and morality.

44. B: When speaking with a patient about sensitive topics, it can be helpful to ask the patient when he is alone and use a quiet, sensitive tone. The CNA should be direct, however, and avoid using clichés or euphemisms. It can also be helpful to use open-ended questions, which gives patients the opportunity to answer for themselves.

45. D: Reflection is the process of listening to what patients say and reflecting it back to them, giving them an opportunity to further explain what they meant. This is the technique used in Choice d. Choice A is an example of showing empathy. Choice B is not helpful for the patient; they may be feeling depressed for reasons that are entirely unrelated to their illness. The response is not sensitive to the patient's needs. Choice C may be appropriate, but shuts down the conversation and the relationship between the patient and the CNA.

46. C: Because of the potential for a patient emergency, it is never appropriate for a CNA to ignore a call bell. She should respond to the bell and see if she is able to assist the patient. Stocking the shelves is not a priority, especially when it comes to patient care. It may be necessary for the CNA to get the assigned aid to help with patient care, but she should verify that nothing urgent is needed first.

47. D: The CNA should never ignore a patient's call bell because it could potentially alert the staff to a dangerous situation. That doesn't mean, however, that the patient has a right to abuse the staff and call bell system. The CNA should establish clear boundaries and expectations about when it is okay to use the call bell. She should also understand that it is quite likely that the patient is anxious or lonely, and should agree to check on her at established intervals. This may help alleviate some of the anxiety. The nurse manager may need to get involved if the above interventions aren't successful.

48. A: The CNA should never take on a patient or task that she does not feel sufficiently trained to handle or comfortable with. She should immediately speak privately with the nurse manager to request additional instructions or training. The CNA should never "just do the best she can" because of the potential for serious complications. Colleagues may be an additional source of information, but the nurse manager should be immediately made aware of the situation, and should be the primary point of contact for the CNA.

49. B: When a sensitive topic is involved, the CNA should utilize the hospital's translation system. This can help the patient feel more comfortable and answer the question more appropriately and accurately. Family members are a good source of assistance for routine tasks and matters that don't involve sensitive topics. Gesturing to the patient in the hope she will understand the question is not a great technique because it can easily lead to misunderstanding. Looking up words on the Internet can be helpful, but will not guarantee that either the patient or the CNA will understand what the other is trying to say.

50. C: Unless the family member has a legal document stating that they are the patient's guardian or holds power of attorney, the patient has a right to privacy. Further, the CNA should not give results to any patient or family member. It's fine to say that the patient seems to be feeling well and offer to get the nurse to discuss details about the test.

51. A: HIPAA guarantees a patient's confidentiality and privacy. It also requires healthcare providers to provide patients with a list of policies that have been designed to protect their privacy. Only providers who are directly caring for someone should have access to their medical chart.

52. B: A CNA should not discuss procedures or what was in the consent forms the patient signed. Only a physician can review and inform a patient of the risks and benefits of having a procedure or treatment. A patient can always withdraw their consent, even if they're about to go into the procedure room. The nurse should notify the physician that the patient has questions so he can arrange to see the patient and discuss her concerns.

53. D: Advanced directives should be promptly placed in the patient's chart and the nurse or physician should be notified. They may need to verify the orders or write new orders for the hospital's order system. Everyone involved in the care of the patient needs to be on the same page and aware of the patient's wishes, even if they are only having a minor procedure.

54. C: A patient has the right to refuse a procedure, even if doing so is not in his best interest. The CNA should explain why frequent turning is important and what may happen if he continues to refuse. Asking what the patient is concerned about or why he doesn't want to be turned can be helpful in identifying solvable problems. If the patient still refuses, the CNA should notify the nurse, who can also speak with the patient and document the incident in the chart.

55. C: All of the choices with the exception of maintenance of personal property are patient responsibilities. Valuable items should be returned to the patient's home or stored with hospital security. Patients should be honest with their caregivers and act in a respectful and appropriate manner. While a patient has the right to refuse treatment, it is expected that they will work with the care team to develop and maintain a mutually acceptable treatment plan.

56. B: A CNA should never administer medication; it's not within her scope of practice. The CNA should go back to the patient and explain that the nurse is with a critical patient and will be with her as soon as possible. Asking another nurse to administer the medication is not an appropriate action because the CNA is then accepting responsibility for delegating the task to another staff member.

57. A: You should refuse to answer the question. The patient has a right to privacy and confidentiality. Even though the colleague cared for the patient in the past, she is not a current, active member of the patient's healthcare team. Therefore, the CNA does not have a right to that information.

58. B: The patient in this situation has a right to respectful care. All patients have the right to receive care, even people injured in the course of committing a crime or those already in the criminal justice system. Patients also have the right to receive care without being discriminated against on the basis of age, gender, nationality, or religion. The right to freedom of choice is the patient's right to have a say in their care plan, and to refuse certain treatments or refuse care altogether.

59. D: A patient absolutely has the right to see his medical chart, but he must follow the procedures put in place by the institution in order to do so. In most cases, the patient will need to contact the medical records department and submit a formal request in writing. The CNA should not provide copies directly to the patient.

60. C: A DNR order is written for a patient so that the health care team involved in his treatment understands what type of emergency care the patient wishes to have should he become incapacitated. It does not release the physician from providing any care, but simply explains the patient's wishes. For example, the patient may not want to be intubated, but may consent to antibiotics or a feeding tube. In most cases, pain management continues to be an important part of a patient's care, even with a DNR order in place. Often, a DNR order is required for patients entering hospice care, but it is not the only reason why a patient would have such an order.

61. C: A CNA could be charged with assault if she threatens or tries to touch a patient (provide care) without the patient's consent. It does not matter if she actually touches the patient or provides the treatment; the patient just needs to be afraid that she will do it. Battery refers to the actual act of touching the patient in a threatening manner or in a way that the patient has not consented to. In the situation outlined in the question, the CNA could be charged with both assault and/or battery, depending on the specific circumstances surrounding the incident.

62. D: The CNA could be charged with negligence because she performed a task in a way that was inconsistent with her training. Only a professional with advanced training or one who needs to maintain a license, such as a doctor or nurse, can be charged with malpractice. A CNA can't because they only need to maintain a certification, not a license. Assault and battery do not apply because the CNA is not behaving in a threatening manner.

63. B: The CNA should follow the chain of command when determining who to report the behavior to. It is inappropriate to contact the physician in charge of the patient's care because he does not have any authority to deal with this type of nursing situation. It is inappropriate to go directly to the nursing supervisor or president of nursing without following the guidelines set in place by the institution.

64. A: The CNA should immediately report the suspected abuse to the charge nurse so she can determine how best to proceed. It is possible that the suspicions have already been addressed, which is why it is not appropriate to directly report the suspected abuse to the police or confront the potential abuser. The behavior should not be ignored, however, because of the potential for the patient being harmed.

65. B: The most important member of the health care team is the patient. His or her needs— medical, spiritual, and emotional—are the most important. The patient must ultimately consent to and be actively involved in their plan of care. What the physician, nurse, and CNA need, recommend, or want takes a back seat to the needs and wishes of the patient.

66. B: The CNA should complete a minimum of 12 hours of continuing education each year to keep her skills up to date. Additional continuing education hours may be necessary, depending on the skill level and needs of the CNA. Her employer should provide some of the continuing education credits, but it is ultimately the responsibility of the CNA to maintain her certification.

67. D: During a code, the CNA should promptly retrieve emergency equipment or other supplies according to the needs of the physicians and nurses. That may include blood from the blood bank, needles, syringes, etc. Documenting the events and administering medications is the responsibility of the nurse, and is outside the scope of practice of the CNA. The CNA should not answer medical questions from the family, but may be able to provide comfort or support if necessary.

68. C: In cases where the patient will be going home to be cared for by the family, it is definitely appropriate for family members to begin to assist in the patient's care. The CNA should allow the daughter to participate in her mother's care, but should be available to supervise and assist as necessary.

69. A: The CNA should prepare the room, ensuring that linens, personal protective equipment, and other medical supplies are present. The CNA should also help orient the patient to the unit and take vital signs. The nurse should complete the admission interview and assessment and coordinate all aspects of care. This includes contacting the pharmacy and ensuring the correct medications are received.

70. C: A serious disagreement with the patient's family is not a reason to refuse an assignment. The CNA must find a way to work professionally with her patient and the family. If the disagreement begins to interfere with the care the patient is receiving, the CNA should speak with her nurse supervisor about the steps that will need to be taken. The other answer choices are all valid reasons for refusing an assignment.

CNA Practice Test #2

1. If a nurse delegates a routine nursing task to a nursing aide, the person who is legally accountable for the patient's safety is which of the following?

    a. Delegating nurse
    b. Nurse aide
    c. Supervisor
    d. Director of nursing

2. How far should a slide sheet extend?

    a. At least from above the head to below the feet
    b. At least from the upper back to the hips
    c. At least from under the head to above the knees
    d. At least from the waist to below the hips

3. If a patient has just had a long-leg plaster cast applied and the cast is still damp, what should the nurse aide do?

    a. Move the cast using the fingertips only
    b. Ensure that the cast is exposed to the air
    c. Cover the cast with a blanket
    d. Avoid pillows under the cast until it's dry

4. Which of the following is an example of a food that is high in protein?

    a. Egg
    b. Banana
    c. Cabbage
    d. Bread

5. If, when assisting a patient to undress, the nurse aide notes bruising and behavior that suggest a patient may be a victim of abuse, what should the nurse aide do?

    a. Ask the patient about it
    b. Stay quiet because there is no proof
    c. Report the concerns to the nurse
    d. Provide the patient with the number of an abuse hotline

6. If planning to use a mechanical lift to move a patient who weighs more than 500 pounds, what is the first thing the nurse aide should do?

    a. Get assistance from another staff member
    b. Ensure that the equipment is in good repair
    c. Explain the procedure to the patient
    d. Check the weight limit for the equipment

7. Which food should a patient on a low-sodium diet avoid?

    a. Egg
    b. Salami
    c. Orange
    d. Spinach

129

8. Which of the following is true for contact precautions?

    a. Gloves are worn for all contact with the patient and the immediate environment

    b. The patient's bed must be separated from another patient's bed by at least 6 feet

    c. The patient's privacy curtain has to be closed only during procedures

    d. The same personal protective equipment (PPE) may be used if caring for two patients in the same room

9. What site is used to check the pulse of a 1-year-old child?

    a. Temporal

    b. Radial

    c. Brachial

    d. Apical

10. After helping a patient onto the toilet, what should be done next?

    a. Watch until the patient finishes

    b. Allow the patient privacy

    c. Stay close but turn away from the patient

    d. Cover the patient's lap with a drape

11. When collecting a stool specimen from a patient, what part of the stool should be collected?

    a. Any part of the stool

    b. Any abnormal-appearing part of the stool

    c. The middle of the stool and any blood, mucus, or abnormality

    d. The end of the stool and any blood, mucus, or abnormality

12. If a patient is to use a cane because of weakness in the left leg, how should the cane be held?

    a. With the tip 12–15 inches to the side of the foot

    b. In either hand that is comfortable

    c. In the left hand

    d. In the right hand

13. If the nurse aide notes that a coworker has spilled water in the hallway when delivering it to a patient, which of the following should the nurse aide do?

    a. Wait until the coworker comes back out and tell the person

    b. Wipe up the spilled water

    c. Call housekeeping to wipe up the water

    d. Tell the nurse that there is spilled water in the hallway

14. If a patient repeatedly asks the nurse aide to repeat what the nurse aide said and turns the volume of the TV up high, what should the nurse aide suspect?

    a. The patient is hard of hearing.

    b. The patient is confused.

    c. The patient is distracted.

    d. The patient is unhappy.

15. When changing the linen on a bed, it's important to do which of the following?

    a. Shake out the sheets to remove any wrinkles
    b. Bring extra linens in case they are needed
    c. Avoid touching the linen to one's uniform
    d. Place the dirty linen on the floor

16. If a patient is having trouble sleeping at night, which of the following should be avoided in the evening?

    a. Coffee
    b. Herbal tea
    c. Orange juice
    d. Sugar candies

17. If the nurse aide needs help from another team member in caring for a patient, an appropriately worded request is

    a. "Can you help me with Room 26A?"
    b. "Can you please help me turn Mrs. Brown in Room 26A for about 5 minutes at 8:30?"
    c. "I need help turning Mrs. Brown. Can you do it?"
    d. "Meet me in Room 26A at 8:30. I need help with the patient."

18. A patient complains of pain in the left leg. What should the nurse aide do?

    a. Palpate the leg to determine where the pain is
    b. Ask the patient to point to the painful areas
    c. Ask the patient which part of the leg hurts
    d. Ask the patient to move the leg around to see if that relieves the pain

19. If a bedbound patient is agitated, angry, and threatening, which of the following should the nurse aide do?

    a. Run out of the room
    b. Tell the patient that the behavior is unacceptable
    c. Stand away from the patient and near the door
    d. Yell for help

20. When the nurse aide is applying elastic compression stockings, where should the patient be?

    a. Lying in bed
    b. Sitting on the side of the bed
    c. Returning to bed
    d. Getting ready to sleep at night

21. A resident in a long-term-care facility has the right to do which of the following?

    a. Bring any personal items that the patient desires
    b. Refuse to allow a roommate in a double room
    c. Swear at staff members
    d. Make complaints about the quality of care

22. Which stool is abnormal and should be reported to the nurse?

    a. Black and tarry stool
    b. Stool with a strong odor
    c. Smooth and soft stool
    d. Dark-brown stool

23. Which of the following is an appropriate documentation of a patient's state of mind?

    a. "Patient crying throughout the morning and refused visitors."
    b. "Patient sad and depressed all morning."
    c. "Patient increasingly withdrawn."
    d. "Patient appears very down and wants no contact with others."

24. A patient is undergoing bladder training to reduce urinary frequency. What does this mean for the patient?

    a. The patient should urinate when feeling the urge.
    b. The patient should delay urinating for as long as possible.
    c. The patient should urinate every hour.
    d. The patient should urinate on a schedule.

25. A patient has scattered personal belongings around the room and bathroom, resulting in a cluttered space. The nurse aide should do which of the following?

    a. Clean up the clutter
    b. Explain that the room looks cluttered
    c. Ask the patient for permission to organize the personal belongings
    d. Remind the patient to organize the personal belongings

26. When assisting a patient with mild to moderate Alzheimer's disease to dress, what should the nurse aide do?

    a. Stack the clothing in the order that the pieces are normally worn
    b. Point out the clothing items one by one as the patient dresses
    c. Lay out all of the clothing separately
    d. Hand the patient one piece of clothing at a time

27. The nurse aide is caring for a home-healthcare patient when the patient's phone rings, and the patient asks the nurse aide to answer the phone. Which of the following is an appropriate telephone greeting?

    a. "Hello, Mrs. Brown's residence."
    b. "Hello."
    c. "Hello, this is Mrs. Brown's home health aide."
    d. "Hello, this is Sally Smith, a home health aide."

28. When preparing a surgical/postoperative bed, what is true of the top linens?

    a. They are folded toward the foot.
    b. They are left off of the bed.
    c. They include extra blankets.
    d. They are folded to one side of the bed.

29. A patient needs to use the bedpan but is too weak to assist the nurse aide. What is the first thing the nurse aide should do after lowering the patient and placing a waterproof pad under the patient?

  a. Flex the patient's knees
  b. Turn the patient to the side facing away from the nurse
  c. Turn the patient to the side facing toward the nurse
  d. Lift the legs and buttocks

30. If a patient asks the nurse aide to explain the purpose of a new medical treatment, which of the following would be the most appropriate response?

  a. "I'll ask your nurse to come in and explain that to you."
  b. "I can't give you that information."
  c. "The purpose is to reduce your episodes of chest pain."
  d. "I don't know what the purpose of the treatment is."

31. If a male patient uses a urinal while in bed, where should the urinal be?

  a. Placed under the covers beside the person
  b. Placed on a bedside stand next to the bed
  c. Placed on the overbed table within easy reach
  d. Attached to a bedrail or urinal holder on a bedrail

32. What should the nurse aide use to cut a patient's fingernails?

  a. Clippers
  b. Scissors
  c. Clippers and a nail file
  d. Scissors and a nail file

33. When transferring a patient from a wheelchair (WC) to a toilet, which of the following is true regarding positioning?

  a. Position the patient's weak side closest to the toilet
  b. Position the WC so it is directly in front of the toilet
  c. Position the WC so it is beside or at a 90° angle to the toilet
  d. Position the patient onto the toilet before loosening the clothing

34. When cleaning the mouth of an unconscious patient, what should the nurse aide use?

  a. A WaterPik
  b. A sponge swab
  c. A soft cloth
  d. A soft toothbrush

35. If a nurse aide turns a patient and discovered that the area over the bony prominence of the right hip is red and irritated, the nurse aide should do which of the following?

  a. Report this observation to the nurse
  b. Massage the area
  c. Apply lotion to the area
  d. Apply a warm compress to the area

36. If a patient's hair is badly tangled and matted, what should the nurse aide do?

    a. Apply hair conditioner to the hair before brushing
    b. Cut out the tangled and matted hair
    c. Brush the hair from the scalp to the hair ends
    d. Brush the hair from the hair ends to the scalp

37. If a nurse aide student is going to observe the nurse aide giving a bed bath to a patient, the nurse aide should do which of the following?

    a. Ask the patient's permission in advance
    b. Tell the patient in advance
    c. Explain that observation is a standard procedure
    d. Pretend that the student is another nurse aide on the unit

38. After bathing a patient, which of the following is used to help prevent friction from two skin surfaces rubbing against each other?

    a. Bath oil
    b. Lotion
    c. Powder
    d. Cream

39. If assisting a patient to brush the teeth, the head of the patient's bed should be elevated to what position?

    a. 75-90°
    b. 45-60°
    c. 30-45°
    d. 20-30°

40. With 24-hour time, how is 3 pm recorded?

    a. 03:00
    b. 30:00
    c. 01:50
    d. 15:00

41. If a patient refuses personal care early in the morning, stating "I'm not a morning person," what should the nurse aide do?

    a. Skip the personal care
    b. Ask the patient when the personal care would be convenient
    c. Insist on providing the personal care
    d. Report the patient to the nurse

42. Which term is used to describe difficulty swallowing?

    a. Dysphagia
    b. Dystonia
    c. Dyspepsia
    d. Dyspnea

43. What is the correct temperature for the water in a basin used for a complete or partial bed bath for a patient?

    a. 98-101 °F
    b. 102-106 °F
    c. 107-110 °F
    d. 110-115 °F

44. If a patient is on a dysphagia diet because of the risk of choking, at least how long should the patient remain sitting upright after eating?

    a. 20 minutes
    b. 40 minutes
    c. 60 minutes
    d. 90 minutes

45. If a nurse asks the nurse aide to deliver a medication to a patient, the nurse aide should do which of the following?

    a. Deliver the medication
    b. Explain that the nurse aide is not allowed to administer medications
    c. Ask what the medication is for before administering it
    d. Make an excuse for why the nurse aide does not have time

46. Which position is recommended to prevent pressure injuries?

    a. 30° lateral
    b. Prone
    c. Full lateral
    d. Sims'

47. If the patient's care plan states "Turn pt. q 2 h," what does this mean?

    a. Turn the patient two times per shift
    b. Turn the patient every 2 hours
    c. Turn the patient with two people
    d. Turn the patient with the bed in the high position

48. If a patient has a feeding tube, the nurse aide may do which of the following?

    a. Reinsert a feeding tube that has been displaced
    b. Check the feeding tube placement
    c. Assist with feedings
    d. Aspirate to determine the residual stomach contents

49. Which of the following is true for lifting a box from the floor?

    a. Keep the back straight and bend at the knees
    b. Bend over at the waist
    c. Use the muscles of the back rather than the legs for lifting
    d. Hold the box away from the body

50. If the nurse aide observes another staff member going through a patient's personal belongs and pocketing an item when the patient is out of the room, what should the nurse aide do?

    a. Assume it is at the patient's request
    b. Confront the staff member
    c. Ignore the situation
    d. Report the observation to a supervisor

51. If the patient's skin sticks to the sheets when the patient slides down in bed, this is referred to as which of the following?

    a. Friction
    b. Shearing
    c. Tearing
    d. Deranging

52. How should a transfer belt be applied?

    a. Over bare skin
    b. Very loosely
    c. When the patient is in a sitting position
    d. With the buckle centered in the front

53. If a patient who weighs 210 pounds must be repositioned toward the head of the bed but can only partially assist with the repositioning, how many staff members are needed?

    a. 1-2
    b. 2-3
    c. 3-4
    d. 4-6

54. If the patient's door is closed when the nurse aide arrives to give morning care, what should the nurse aide do?

    a. Enter quietly so as not to disturb the patient
    b. Knock before entering the room
    c. Assume that the patient does not want to be disturbed
    d. Return at a later time

55. What is the most effective way to prevent the spread of healthcare-associated infections, such as *Clostridium difficile* or methicillin-resistant *Staphylococcus aureus*?

    a. Wear face masks
    b. Wear gowns when in patients' rooms
    c. Limit time with patients
    d. Use proper hand hygiene

56. If a patient refuses to get out of a chair and the nurse aide grasps the patient around the waist and forcibly removes the patient from the chair, what could this be considered?

    a. Abuse
    b. A boundary violation
    c. Battery
    d. Negligence

57. When washing the hands with soap and water, the nurse aide should lather the hands for at least how long?

    a. 30 seconds
    b. 20 seconds
    c. 10 seconds
    d. 5 seconds

58. Which of the following is part of a safety check?

    a. Ensuring that adaptive devices are stored in a closet or cabinet.
    b. Ensuring that the bed is locked in the high position.
    c. Ensuring that hearing aids are sent home so they don't get lost.
    d. Ensuring that the patient's water and call bell are within reach.

59. If a patient has violent restraints in place, what is the minimum frequency they must be checked on?

    a. Every 5 minutes
    b. Every 15 minutes
    c. Every 30 minutes
    d. Every 60 minutes

60. The nurse aide is taking routine vital signs for a 70-year-old patient. Which of the following should immediately be reported to the nurse?

    a. BP 176/100
    b. Pulse 88
    c. Respirations 14
    d. Temperature 38 °C

61. If a patient is being monitored for intake and output and drinks 6 ounces of apple juice, what is this equal to?

    a. 90 mL
    b. 120 mL
    c. 180 mL
    d. 240 mL

62. Which position has the patient on their left side with their right leg flexed so that their left arm and leg are behind them?

    a. Lateral
    b. Prone
    c. Supine
    d. Sims'

63. If a sign on a patient's door says "NPO," what does this mean?

    a. The patient is not to be disturbed.
    b. The patient is nonambulatory.
    c. The patient is nonhearing.
    d. The patient is to have nothing by mouth.

64. What is the normal range for oral temperature?
  a. 35.9-37 °C (96.6-98.6 °F)
  b. 36.5-37.5 °C (97.6-99.6 °F)
  c. 37.0-38.1 °C (98.6-100.6 °F)
  d. 38-39 °C (100.4-102.2 °F)

65. If a patient is to maintain abduction after a left hip replacement, how should the patient be positioned?
  a. With the legs apart
  b. With the legs close together
  c. With the left leg elevated
  d. With the knee flexed on the left leg

66. Which of the following is true for the nurse aide when carrying out range-of-motion (ROM) exercises?
  a. Move the joint to the point of pain
  b. Force the joint slightly past its normal range
  c. Move the joint slowly and gently
  d. Move the joint quickly and forcefully

67. A person dying of cancer is withdrawn and refusing food, stating, "What's the point?" Which of the following is the most appropriate response?
  a. "I know how you feel."
  b. "If you'd like to talk, I'll listen."
  c. "Try to concentrate on the good things in your life."
  d. "You may still have weeks of life ahead if you eat."

68. A Muslim patient has been admitted to a long-term-care facility and is nonverbal after a stroke. What should the nurse aide anticipate that the patient will probably want to avoid eating?
  a. Beef
  b. Fish
  c. Poultry
  d. Pork

69. An older adult patient is recovering from major surgery, and the nurse aide notices that the patient has become slightly confused and increasingly agitated. How should the nurse aide respond?
  a. Report this to the nurse immediately
  b. Tell the patient to calm down
  c. Ask the patient what is wrong
  d. Assume that this is a normal postoperative condition

70. What type of precautions should the nurse aide should use in caring for a patient who is human immunodeficiency virus (HIV) positive?
  a. Contact
  b. Standard
  c. Droplet
  d. Airborne

Answer Key and Explanations for Test #2

1. A: If a nurse delegates a routine nursing task to a nursing aide, the person who is legally accountable for the patient's safety is the delegating nurse. The nurse determines whether the task is within the range of functions of the nursing aide in their state and whether the task can be safely delegated. The nurse must consider the needs of the patient, the extent of the task, and the nursing aide's abilities.

2. C: A slide sheet should extend at least from under the head to above the knees. The purpose of a slide sheet is to move the patient while avoiding the risk of friction and shear. If using the draw sheet (which extends below the head) to move a patient, then one person should support the head and neck. The patient can flex the knees to assist with repositioning, if able to do so.

3. B: If a patient has just had a long-leg plaster cast applied and it is still damp, the nurse aide should ensure that the cast is exposed to the air so it can dry thoroughly. No blankets should be placed over the cast until it is completely dry. A fan may be used to speed drying. Pillows should be placed under the length of the cast, and the nurse aide should use only the flat part of the palms to move the cast rather than the fingertips, which may leave indentations.

4. A: An example of a food that is high in protein is an egg. Other high-protein foods include meat products, soy products (such as tofu), and nuts. Beans are high in protein, but they are also high in carbohydrates. All vegetables and fruits are high in carbohydrates, but they also contain vitamins, minerals, and fiber that are essential for nutrition. Bread and desserts are especially high in carbohydrates, and many have little nutritional value.

5. C: If, when assisting a patient to undress, the nursing aide notes bruising and behavior that suggest the patient may be a victim of abuse, the nursing aide should report the concerns to the nurse. The nurse can then follow up with an examination and interview and offer assistance to the patient if it appears warranted, although many abuse victims deny that they are being abused.

6. D: If planning to use a mechanical lift to move a patient who weighs 500 pounds (morbidly obese), the first thing the nurse aide should do is to check the weight limit for the equipment. Most standard lifts can support weight up to 450 pounds, but bariatric equipment that can support 500-1,000 pounds may be necessary for patients who are extremely heavy. If the mechanical lift cannot support the weight, the patient may fall and be injured. The nurse aide should never operate a lift alone; therefore, getting assistance from another staff member is also important once the appropriate lift is obtained.

7. B: A patient on a low-sodium diet should avoid foods that are high in salt (sodium chloride), such as salami. All processed meats (bologna, hot dogs, corned beef, pastrami) are high in sodium. Low-sodium foods include virtually all fruits and vegetables. Most lean meats are low in sodium. The patient should avoid foods with added salt, such as many canned foods and frozen prepared meals, and should avoid the sauces that sometimes come with frozen vegetables.

8. A: For contact precautions, gloves are worn for all contact with the patient and the immediate environment. Contact precautions are used for infections that are spread by touch, such as *Clostridium difficile*. A gown is required for direct contact with the patient or potentially contaminated environmental surfaces, such as the bed and bedside stand. PPE should not be reused or used with more than one patient, even if the patient is in the same room.

9. D: Although the radial artery in the wrist is the site most often used to measure the pulse rate, for children younger than 2 years of age, the apical site is used, auscultating the rate with a stethoscope. The pulse is auscultated at the fourth intercostal space, left midclavicular line (the midpoint of the left side of the chest). In adults, the apical pulse is auscultated at the fifth intercostal space.

10. B: After helping a patient onto the toilet, it's important to allow the patient privacy. If safe to do so, the nurse aide should wait outside of the bathroom and close the door while making sure the patient has access to a call bell and staying close at hand to be available for when the patient has finished toileting. If the patient is using a commode, the patient should be placed behind curtains or a screen so they cannot be seen if someone opens the door to the room.

11. C: When collecting a stool specimen from a patient, the specimen should be taken from the middle of the stool and from any area with blood, mucus, or other abnormality. The nurse aide should place the specimen pan on the back of the toilet/commode so that the front part of the toilet is free. The nurse should caution the patient to try to avoid urinating into the specimen container. The patient may urinate first before the specimen container is placed if comfortable doing so. To collect the specimen, a tongue blade or spoon attached to a stool specimen container lid is used.

12. D: If a patient is to use a cane because of weakness in the left leg, the patient should hold the cane in the right hand. When the patient is standing in neutral position, the elbow should be bent at approximately a 15° angle so that the arm can straighten when the cane is advanced. The cane is usually placed approximately 6-10 inches beside the foot because the patient's gait will not be stable if the cane is held too far to the side.

13. B: If the nurse aide notes that a coworker has spilled water in the hallway when delivering it to a patient, the nurse aide should wipe up the spilled water as soon as possible because it poses an immediate safety risk to others walking in the hallway. As a team member, the nurse aide should be willing to help out other members of the staff without worrying about whose responsibility the problem is.

14. A: If a patient repeatedly asks the nurse aide to repeat what the nurse aide said and turns the volume of the TV up high, the nurse aide should suspect that the patient is hard of hearing. The nurse aide should alert the nurse. If the patient has hearing aids, the nurse aide should make sure that they have functioning batteries and are securely in place in the patient's ears.

15. C: When changing linen on the bed, it's important to avoid touching the linen to one's uniform because the linen is considered dirty, so it should be held away from the uniform. Shaking linens can spread microbes. Linen should be placed on the bed and unfolded, piece by piece. Dirty linen should never be placed on the floor, but instead in the dirty linen receptacle. Any extra linen that is not used is considered dirty and cannot then be used for another patient.

16. A: If a patient is having trouble sleeping at night, the patient should avoid drinking coffee in the evening because it is high in caffeine, a stimulant. Other foods or drinks high in caffeine include cola and many other carbonated drinks, chocolate, energy drinks, and tea (black and green). Herbal tea is usually decaffeinated and is not actually made from tea leaves.

17. B: If the nurse aide needs help from another team member in caring for a patient, an appropriate request is "Can you please help me turn Mrs. Brown in Room 26A for about 5 minutes at 8:30?" When making a request, the nurse aide should remember to say "please" and should be specific about the type of help, when it's needed, and the expected duration. Patients should never be referred to by their room number instead of by name.

18. B: If a patient complains of pain in the left leg, the nurse aide should ask the patient to point to the painful areas so that the nurse aide can better describe the pain to the nurse. The nurse aide may ask general questions such as "When did the pain start?" and "How painful is it on a scale of 1 to 10?" but should not palpate the leg or ask the patient to move the leg around because the nurse should carry out that assessment.

19. C: If a bedbound patient is agitated, angry, and threatening, the nurse aide should stand away from the patient and near the door, especially if the patient has access to items that could be thrown. The nurse aide should speak calmly and quietly, trying to calm the patient. The nurse aide should leave the room as soon possible and report the patient's behavior to the nurse. If the patient is ambulatory, the nurse aide should leave immediately to avoid harm.

20. A: When the nurse aide is applying elastic compression stockings, the patient should be lying in bed. Compression stockings are worn when the patient is out of bed in a chair or walking to reduce swelling in the legs. The stockings should be removed when the patient goes back to bed, and they are not worn at night. Compression stockings cannot be properly fitted if swelling is already present (which can be induced if a patient is sitting on the side of the bed with their legs dangling).

21. D: A resident in a long-term-care facility has the right to make complaints about the quality of care. The Older Americans Act established an ombudsman program to identify, investigate, and find a solution to complaints made by patients or on behalf of patients who are unable to do so on their own. Any patient who asks to file a complaint should be assisted to contact someone from the ombudsman program. Most facilities limit the personal belongings that a patient can bring; for example, they may prohibit weapons.

22. A: Normal stools may vary in color and consistency, but a black, tarry stool is abnormal and should be reported to the nurse because it may indicate that the patient has bleeding in the upper gastrointestinal system. Blood appears black when it has been digested. Iron preparations and medications that contain bismuth may also cause the stool to appear black. Additionally, some foods, such as black licorice and beets, may make the stool appear black.

23. A: An appropriate documentation of a patient's state of mind is "Patient crying throughout the morning and refused visitors." This is an objective statement of what was actually observed, not a subjective interpretation of what the nurse aide thinks the behavior indicates ("withdrawn," "down," "sad," or "depressed"). The nurse aide must always try to be as factual as possible when documenting.

24. D: If a patient is undergoing bladder training to reduce urinary frequency, the patient should urinate on a schedule. The registered nurse will assign the schedule, usually every 2-3 hours, depending on how frequently the patient has been urinating. The patient should try to wait until the scheduled time to void if it can be done without discomfort or incontinence. Over time, the duration is extended.

25. C: If a patient has scattered personal belongings around the room and bathroom, resulting in a cluttered space, the nurse aide should ask the patient for permission to organize the personal belongings. The nurse aide should not handle any personal belongings without permission and should insist on moving items only if they pose a safety hazard, such as when items are placed on the floor.

26. A: When assisting a patient with mild to moderate Alzheimer's disease to dress, the nurse aide should encourage the patient to be as independent as possible and should stack the clothing in the order that the pieces are normally worn. For example, the undergarments (panties, bra, shorts, undershirt) should be on top of the stack. This allows the patient to work down the stack without getting confused about the order.

27. B: If the nurse aide is caring for a home-healthcare patient when the patient's phone rings, and the patient asks the nurse aide to answer the phone, an appropriate telephone greeting is "Hello." Because the nurse aide can't know who is calling, giving out the patient's name is not appropriate. The nurse aide is violating confidentiality if identifying as a home health aide because this is telling the caller that the patient is in need of medical care.

28. D: When preparing a surgical/postoperative bed, the top linens are folded to one side of the bed because the patient will be moved onto the bed from a stretcher. If a patient is returning to the bed after surgery, a complete linen change should be done in preparation for the patient's return. If the patient is going for a treatment via stretcher and will return to the bed, the bed should be prepared with the top linens to the side, but a complete linen change is not necessary.

29. B: If a patient needs to use the bedpan but is too weak to assist the nurse aide, the first thing the nurse aide should do after lowering the patient and placing a waterproof pad under the patient is to turn the patient to the side facing away from the nurse. The nurse aide holds the bedpan up against the buttocks, centering it and ensuring that it is back far enough, and then rolls the patient back onto the bedpan. The head of the bed should be raised to Fowler's position or a position of comfort.

30. A: If a patient asks the nurse aide to explain the purpose of a new medical treatment, the most appropriate response is, "I'll ask your nurse to come in and explain that to you." Explaining medical treatments is within the scope of practice of the nurse and not within the range of functions of the nurse aide, so even when the nurse aide knows the purpose, the explanation should be left to the nurse who should be better prepared to answer questions about the treatment.

31. D: If a male patient uses a urinal while in bed, the urinal should be attached to a bedrail or urinal holder on a bedrail. If the patient doesn't want the urinal to be seen, it can be covered with a small towel. The urinal should not be placed under the covers because the patient may roll onto it, and it should never be placed on a surface that may contain food or drinks, such as a bedside stand or overbed table.

32. C: To cut a patient's fingernails, the nurse aide should use clippers (to cut the straight across) and a nail file (to smooth and round the edges). The nurse aide should not cut the nails with scissors. The nurse aide must first get approval for cutting a patient's nails because some patients require a specialist to do so (particularly patients with diabetes). Before cutting the nails, the patient should wash the hands and soak the fingernails to soften them. The nurse aide should check for abnormal nails (thick, discolored, or cracked) and hangnails.

33. C: When transferring a patient from a wheelchair (WC) to a toilet, position the WC so it is beside or at a 90° angle to the toilet because these positions make it easier to transfer the patient. The clothing should be loosened before the transfer but lowered after the patient is on the toilet. The patient's strong side should be closest to the toilet so that the patient can assist with the transfer more easily.

34. B: When cleaning the mouth of an unconscious patient, the nurse aide should use a sponge swab. The patient should be placed in a side-lying position facing the nurse aide with a towel under the patient's face and upper chest. The teeth should be separated with a plastic tongue depressor (wood might chip or break if the patient bites down) and the swab, dampened with a cleaning agent, is gently inserted into the mouth to clean all tooth surfaces, the tongue, the roof of the mouth, and the insides of the cheeks.

35. A: If a nurse aide turns a patient and discovers that the area over the bony prominence of the right hip is red and irritated, the nurse aide should report this observation to the nurse who can evaluate the patient's skin and advise the nurse aide of the next steps. The patient should be positioned so that no pressure is applied to this area because the patient may be developing a pressure injury.

36. D: If a patient's hair is badly tangled and matted, the nurse aide should brush the hair from the hair ends to the scalp, loosening the tangles and matted hair with as little force as possible. Though tempting, the nurse aide should never cut any of the patient's hair, even if the patient asks that the nurse aide do so. Only a licensed beautician can cut a patient's hair and only with permission of the patient or the patient's representative.

37. A: If a nurse aide student is going to observe the nurse aide giving a bed bath to a patient, the nurse aide should ask the patient's permission in advance and should respect the patient's wishes and any limitations that the patient requests. Even though teaching hospitals typically include the fact that patients may be observed by students in the notice of privacy practices, patients' wishes should still be respected as much as possible.

38. C: After bathing a patient, powder can be used to help prevent friction from two skin surfaces rubbing against each other. Areas that are often powdered include under the breasts, under abdominal folds, between the buttocks, and under the arms. Care must be taken to avoid the vaginal area or a heavy layer of powder because it may become caked and irritating, especially if the patient perspires a lot.

39. A: If assisting a patient to brush the teeth, the head of the patient's bed should be elevated to 75-90° because this lessens the chance that the patient could choke on fluid running down the throat. The nurse aide should place a towel on the patient's chest, dampen the toothbrush, apply toothpaste, and then gently brush all surfaces of the teeth, the top of the tongue, and the roof of the mouth (avoiding the back of the mouth because this may trigger the gag reflex). The patient then rinses the mouth and spits into the kidney-shaped basin.

40. D: With 24-hour time, 3 pm is recorded as 15:00. Twenty four-hour time is recorded with four digits, so 1 through 9 are preceded by a zero. The time begins at midnight (00:00 or 24:00) and increases by 1:00 each hour, so 7 am is 07:00. For afternoon times, the easiest way to translate standard time into 24-hour time is to start with 12:00 (noon) and add 1:00 for each hour, so 3 pm is 12:00 plus 3:00 which equals 15:00.

41. B: If a patient refuses personal care early in the morning, stating "I'm not a morning person," the nurse aide should ask the patient when the personal care would be convenient and try to accommodate the patient's wishes as much as possible. If the nurse aide has a busy schedule, the nurse aide may suggest options, such as "How about 9:30 or 10:00?" Although patients have the right to refuse care, the nurse aide should still try to come to a compromise with the patient and provide the necessary care.

42. A: Dysphagia is the term used to describe difficulty swallowing. Dystonia is involuntary muscle contractions that cause twisting of body parts or repetitive movements. Dyspepsia is indigestion, which may be caused by food or medications. Dyspnea is difficulty breathing. The prefix *dys-* in a word usually carries the meanings of bad, difficult, or painful.

43. D: The correct temperature for the water in a basin used for a complete or partial bed bath for a patient is 110-115 °F. Note that this is a higher temperature than what is used for a tub bath or shower (usually approximately 105 °F) because the water in a basin tends to lose temperature

143

rapidly during the bathing process. When first starting the bath, check to make sure that the damp washcloth is not too hot for the patient.

44. C: If a patient is on a dysphagia diet because of the risk of choking, the patient should remain sitting upright after eating for at least 60 minutes. This reduces the risk of esophageal reflux, which can result in aspiration. Dysphagia is difficulty swallowing and may occur with a number of disorders, including stroke, Parkinson's disease, multiple sclerosis, muscular dystrophy, and cancers of the throat.

45. B: If a nurse asks the nurse aide to deliver a medication to a patient, the nurse aide should explain that they are not allowed to administer medications because it is clearly outside of the range of functions permitted to nurse aides. The nurse aide should remain polite but firm in refusing to deliver the medication because doing so could increase risk to the patient and could result in disciplinary action or loss of employment for the nurse aide.

46. A: The position that is recommended to prevent pressure injuries is the 30° lateral position. In this position, the pressure is on the fleshy portion of the buttocks rather than the bony prominence. The patient's knees should be flexed, and a pillow is placed under the head, between the leg, and along the back (a back wedge can also be used). Another pillow may be placed under the upper arm if needed for comfort.

47. B: If the patient's care plan states "Turn pt. q 2 h," this means to turn the patient every 2 hours. Common abbreviations include the following:

ac = before meals	Dx = diagnosis
pc = after meals	Hx = history
BID = twice daily	w or c̄ = with
TID = 3× daily	w/o or s̄ = without
QID = 4× daily	BP = blood pressure
HS = hour of sleep	NPO = nothing by mouth (nil per os)
q = every (q 4 h)	VS = vital signs (BP, TPR)
c/o = complains of	hr = hour(s)
stat = immediately	prn = as needed

48. C: If a patient has a feeding tube, the nurse aide may assist with feedings under the direction of the nurse. However, the nurse aide cannot do skilled nursing procedures, such as inserting a feeding tube, checking the feeding tube placement, or aspirating to determine the patient's residual stomach contents. If a feeding is inadvertently administered into the lungs, the patient may develop severe aspiration pneumonia.

49. A: If lifting a box from the floor, the nurse aide should keep the back straight, the feet at least 12 inches (or shoulder width) apart, bend at the knees (squat), and use the muscles in the legs to lift the box rather than the muscles of the back. The nurse aide should hold the box close to the body. Heavy lifting (including items, equipment, and patients) should be avoided if at all possible because it is a leading cause of back injuries to healthcare workers.

50. D: If the nurse aide observes another staff member going through a patient's personal belongs and pocketing an item when the patient is out of the room, the nurse aide should report the observation to a supervisor. Investigation and disciplinary actions are the supervisor's responsibility if a problem arises. The nurse aide should not confront another staff member unless what the staff member is doing is putting the patient at risk, such as if a staff member is abusing a patient.

51. B: If the patient's skin sticks to the sheets when the patient slides down in bed, this is referred to as shearing. Shearing causes injury to deep tissues because the pressure on the tissue causes the surface tissue to stay adhered to the sheet and the tissue underneath to separate and tear. Shearing is one of the leading causes of tissue breakdown and pressure ulcers. Shearing is often combined with friction, increasing damage to the tissues.

52. C: A transfer belt should be applied when the patient is in a sitting position; it should always be applied over clothing and not against bare skin because it may cause irritation. The belt should be snug but not uncomfortable and with the buckle off-center in the front or the back. For female patients, the nurse aide should make sure that the breasts are not directly under the belt, especially if the patient has pendulous breasts.

53. C: If a patient weighs more than 200 pounds and must be repositioned toward the head of the bed but can only partially assist with the repositioning, the number of staff members needed is three to four. If the patient weighs less than 200 pounds and can only partially assist with the repositioning, two to three people are needed. If a patient is completely unable to assist, a mechanical lift may be indicated unless the patient is very lightweight.

54. B: If the patient's door is closed when the nurse aide arrives to give morning care, the nurse aide should knock before entering the room. Mornings tend to be noisy times, so the patient will likely be awake or have to awaken for breakfast, and the patient may have closed the door to keep the noise down. In some cases, staff members may have closed the door as well during the night to avoid disturbing the patient, so a closed door doesn't always mean that the patient does not want to be disturbed.

55. D: The most effective way to prevent the spread of healthcare-associated infections, such as *Clostridium difficile* or methicillin-resistant *Staphylococcus aureus*, is to use proper hand hygiene, including hand washing and the use of an alcohol-based sanitizing rub, before and after contact with each patient. Most healthcare-associated infections are spread through contact, so standard and contact precautions are essential in controlling the spread of infections.

56. C: If a patient refuses to get out of a chair and the nurse aide grasps the patient around the waist and forcibly removes the patient from the chair, this could be considered battery. Threatening or attempting to touch a person without the person's permission is assault, so assault and battery often go together. It's important to get a patient's permission even though this may be difficult if the patient is confused. If the patient will not cooperate, the nurse aide should ask the nurse for assistance.

57. B: When washing the hands with soap and water, the nurse aide should lather the hands for at least 20 seconds. Washing the hands should include the area extending 3-4 inches above the wrists. The hands should always be kept below the elbows while washing and should not touch any part of the sink. The nails are cleaned by rubbing them against the palm of the opposite hand.

58. D: A safety check includes ensuring that the patient's water and call bell are within reach. The bed should be in a low position and the siderails should be up or down according to the patient's care plan. Adaptive devices, such as hearing aids, glasses, walkers, and canes, should be within reach or easily accessible by the patient. The floor in the room and pathway to the bathroom should be uncluttered and unobstructed to reduce the risk of falls.

59. B: If a patient has violent restraints in place (indicated when the patient is actively violent toward the staff or self), the patient must be checked on at least every 15 minutes. Nonviolent restraints are indicated for confused/disoriented patients who are putting themselves or others at risk (such as mildly sedated and intubated patients who are reaching for their endotracheal tube or confused patients who are pulling out their IV or nasogastric tubes), and they must be checked on every 2 hours. A physician's order is required for the use of any type of restraint, and other restraint alternatives, such as treating pain or comforting the patient, must be tried before restraints are applied. The least restrictive restraints should be used and for the shortest possible length of time. Restraints may not be used for staff convenience or discipline, but they may be used to protect the safety of the patient or others.

60. A: If the nurse aide is taking routine vital signs for a 70-year-old patient, the vital sign that should be immediately reported to the nurse is BP of 176/100. The upper limits of normal are 140/90, so anything higher is a cause for concern, especially if this is a new finding. A sudden elevation of BP increases the risk that the patient may have a stroke. The nurse needs to assess the patient to try to determine the cause of the high blood pressure.

61. C: If a patient is being monitored for intake and output and drinks 6 ounces of apple juice, this is equal to 180 mL. In healthcare, the metric system is typically used instead of the imperial system (which includes ounces, pounds, inches, and feet) because the metric system is more precise and allows for easier measurement of small quantities, weights, and volumes. The Celsius scale, used for temperatures, is also part of the metric system, and it uses 0 as the freezing point.

62. D: If a patient is on the left side with the right leg flexed so the left arm and leg are behind the patient, this position is the Sims' (aka left Sims') position. The patient is generally placed in the Sims' position for procedures (such as enemas) more than in the lateral position, during which one leg is typically on top of the other. The prone position is the patient with the abdomen down, and the supine position is the patient flat on the back.

63. D: If a sign on a patient's door says "NPO" (from Latin *nil per os*), this means nothing by mouth. Patients may be restricted from food and drink for 6-12 hours before surgery or other procedures. The nurse aide should remind the patient and any guests or family members present that the patient cannot eat or drink because doing so increases the risk of aspiration if the patient is anesthetized and may interfere with some testing results.

64. B: The normal range for oral temperature is 36.5-37.5 °C. Temperature chart (normal range):

Site	Fahrenheit	Celsius
Axillary	96.6-98.6 °F	35.9-37.0 °C
Oral	97.6-99.6 °F	36.5-37.5 °C
Rectal	98.6-100.6 °F	37.0-38.1 °C
Temporal	99.6 °F	37.5 °C
Tympanic membrane	98.6 °F	37.0 °C

65. A: If a patient is to maintain abduction after a left hip replacement, this means that the patient should be positioned with the legs apart. Usually, a pillow is placed between the patient's legs when the patient is in bed as a reminder to maintain the correct position. The opposite of abduction (away from the midline of the body) is adduction (toward the midline of the body).

66. C: When carrying out range-of-motion (ROM) exercises, the nurse aide should move the joint slowly and gently. The purpose of ROM exercises is to maintain function and to prevent contractures (such as after a stroke or injury), so the joint should not be forced past its normal range or to the point where it is painful. ROM exercises should be carried out on the joints as directed by the nurse, so not all patients will have ROM exercises performed on all joints.

67. B: If a person dying of cancer is withdrawn and refusing food, stating, "What's the point?" the most appropriate response is, "If you'd like to talk, I'll listen." The nurse aide should avoid making statements such as "I know how you feel" because that is likely not true and patients facing death may have a hard time looking at the positives or contemplating their life ahead. Encouraging patients to express their feelings may help to reduce some anxiety.

68. D: Muslim and Jewish patients often want to avoid eating pork because of religious restrictions, although what is true for the religion may not always hold true for the individual. Sometimes, family members are able to provide information about dietary restrictions if a patient is nonverbal and unable to communicate. Even if a patient is unaware of their surroundings, their religious beliefs should still be respected.

69. A: If an older adult patient is recovering from major surgery and the nurse aide notices that the patient has become slightly confused and agitated, the nurse aide should immediately report this to the nurse. Especially in an older adult, these may be signs of delirium. Other signs may include slow movement, drowsiness, incontinence, incoherent speech, and emotional changes. With delirium, symptoms may fluctuate.

70. B: If a patient is HIV positive, the nurse aide should use standard precautions. HIV does not spread through casual contact but rather through contact with body fluids, such as blood. Standard precautions must be used with all patients and includes wearing appropriate PPE when exposed to patients' bodily fluids. PPE may include gloves, gown, and face protection (goggles, mask, and shield). Standard precautions include appropriate hand hygiene and respiratory hygiene.

CNA Practice Test #3

1. If a patient is to use crutches because of no weight bearing on one leg, what type of gait will the patient use?

    a. Two-point

    b. Three-point

    c. Four-point

    d. Swing-to

2. A home health nurse aide is caring for a patient and inadvertently receives a needlestick injury with a used insulin syringe. Which of the following is true regarding this situation?

    a. The nurse aide need not worry about it because diabetes is not contagious.

    b. The nurse aide should expect to have to pay for any testing needed.

    c. The nurse aide has no right to refuse testing for human immunodeficiency virus.

    d. The nurse aide should report the exposure to the home health agency immediately.

3. Before obtaining a sputum specimen, the nurse aide should ask the patient to do which of the following?

    a. Rinse their mouth with mouthwash

    b. Rinse their mouth with water

    c. Expectorate (spit) into a kidney basin

    d. To avoid drinking fluids for 30 minutes

4. If a patient has been incontinent of urine in bed, which of the following is an appropriate response?

    a. "You should have called for help earlier."

    b. "I'm sorry, you must be so embarrassed."

    c. "Let me help you get clean right away."

    d. "Why did you wet your bed?"

5. Standard precautions include which of the following?

    a. Wearing personal protective equipment (PPE) when in contact with blood or body fluids

    b. Wearing gloves for all patient contact

    c. Reusing the same PPE for the same patient

    d. Keeping at least 6 feet between patients' beds

6. Where do pressure injuries most often occur?

    a. In fatty tissue

    b. In muscle tissue

    c. In obese adults

    d. Over bony prominences

7. A patient is to drink 1 liter of water as part of the prep for a colonoscopy. What is this volume equivalent to?

    a. 500 mL

    b. 1,000 mL

    c. 1,200 mL

    d. 1,800 mL

8. Approximately how much sleep do school-age children (6–12 years old) need?
   a. 11–14 hours per day
   b. 10–13 hours per day
   c. 9–12 hours per day
   d. 8–10 hours per day

9. If a patient has just received an oral pain medication, how long should the nurse aide wait before assisting the patient to get up into a chair?
   a. 5–10 minutes
   b. 20–30 minutes
   c. 40–50 minutes
   d. 60–90 minutes

10. If changing a front-opening gown while the patient is in bed, what is the first step?
   a. Undue the fasteners (buttons, zippers, ties)
   b. Help the patient to sit up
   c. Slide the gown off of the shoulders
   d. Pull the bottom of the gown up toward the chest

11. Over what time period should a cleansing enema (500–1,000 mL) be administered?
   a. 2–3 minutes
   b. 5–10 minutes
   c. 10–15 minutes
   d. 15–20 minutes

12. If a patient wears disposable incontinence briefs for urinary and fecal incontinence, how often should the nurse aide provide perineal care?
   a. After each episode of incontinence
   b. After each episode of fecal incontinence
   c. Every 3 hours
   d. When there is obvious soiling or irritation

13. Before bedtime, which of the following may help to relax a patient so that the patient can sleep better?
   a. Cup of hot tea
   b. Hot shower
   c. Physical exercise
   d. Gentle back massage

14. A nurse aide notices that a patient assigned to another nurse aide is trying to drink water but is having difficulty raising the glass. What should the nurse aide do?
   a. Notify the patient's nurse aide
   b. Offer to assist the patient
   c. Let the patient continue to try to drink the water
   d. Tell the nurse

15. What condition is required for a nurse aide to carry out a delegated task?

    a. If the task is within the nurse aide's range of functions
    b. If a nurse has delegated the task
    c. If the task has been done by other nurse aides
    d. If the nurse aide is familiar with the task

16. If the healthcare organization uses electronic health records to document patient care, what should the nurse aide do?

    a. Write the personal username and password on a card and carry it in a pocket
    b. Allow others to use the personal username and password if they have forgotten their own
    c. Guard the personal username and password from everyone else
    d. Only allow nurses and physicians to use the personal password and username

17. Which electronic communication to a friend is acceptable under the Health Insurance Portability and Accountability Act of 1996 for a nurse aide working in home health care?

    a. "Can you pick me up at my last patient's home at 2600 Roc Avenue?"
    b. "Look at this picture of my patient and me!"
    c. "My patient, Sally Brown, is my age."
    d. "My last patient of the day lives near Pizza Palace, so I'll meet you there."

18. To use proper body mechanics, the nurse aide should avoid which of the following?

    a. Stretching overhead more than 20 inches to reach items
    b. Lifting with the leg muscles rather than with the back muscles
    c. Flexing at the hips and knees rather than at the waist
    d. Pushing rather than pulling heavy items

19. Typically, how times per week do older adults typically need a complete bath?

    a. One
    b. Two
    c. Five
    d. Seven

20. Before shaving a male patient's face with a safety razor, which of the following should the nurse aide do first?

    a. Wash his face with soap and water
    b. Apply soap to the face
    c. Apply a warm, moist cloth to the face
    d. Apply talcum powder to the face

21. If using a shampoo cap to wash a patient's hair, what is the first step?

    a. Warm the cap
    b. Comb or brush the hair
    c. Wet the hair
    d. Place the cap on the patient's head

22. What role does the nurse aide serve as part of a team in the nursing process?
   a. Developing goals
   b. Assessing progress
   c. Assessing medical needs
   d. Reporting observations

23. A patient with Alzheimer's disease insists on carrying a baby doll with her at all times and talks to the doll as though it is a real person. What should the nurse aide do?
   a. Tell the patient that the doll isn't a real person
   b. Ensure that the patient always has the doll
   c. Put the doll away out of sight
   d. Tell the patient that she's lucky to have such a good baby

24. When is a stand-pivot transfer appropriate?
   a. If the patient can assist with the transfer
   b. If the patient is lightweight
   c. If the patient is unable to bear weight
   d. If the patient is of a heavier weight

25. If a patient's son asks the nurse aide why the patient is no longer receiving physical therapy, how should the nurse aide respond?
   a. Explain that the patient wasn't showing progress
   b. Explain that the nurse aide isn't qualified to answer
   c. Refer the son to the nurse for information
   d. Deny any knowledge of the reason

26. If a patient's oxygen saturation per pulse oximeter has been 95%–97% consistently but suddenly drops to 78% and the patient shows no signs of respiratory distress, the nurse aide should immediately do which of the following?
   a. Tell the nurse
   b. Sit the patient upright
   c. Assess the patient's respiratory status
   d. Reposition the pulse oximeter

27. Which of the following observations must be immediately reported to the nurse?
   a. Patient shows improvement in ambulation.
   b. Patient reports a sudden loss of vision in one eye.
   c. Patient complains of slight muscle soreness after physical therapy.
   d. Patient reports sleeping poorly because of noise and interruptions during the night.

28. How often should bedbound patients be repositioned?
   a. At least every 1–2 hours
   b. At least every 2–3 hours
   c. At least every 3–4 hours
   d. At least every 4–5 hours

29. Which directional term is used to describe the body part closest to the center or to the point of attachment, such as the upper arm rather than the lower?

  a. Anterior
  b. Posterior
  c. Proximal
  d. Distal

30. When reporting to a nurse about an older adult patient, how should the nurse aide address the patient?

  a. By first name
  b. By title and last name
  c. By a term of endearment
  d. By room and bed number

31. If a procedure needs to be done "stat," what does this mean?

  a. At bedtime
  b. As needed
  c. As soon as possible
  d. Immediately

32. A long-term-care patient does not want to participate in group activities. Which of the following should the nurse aide do?

  a. Ask what the patient would prefer to do
  b. Insist that the patient participate in the activities
  c. Explain that group activities are important
  d. Ask the patient to explain the reason for the refusal to participate

33. If a patient slips and falls onto the floor during a transfer but appears uninjured, what should the nurse aide do?

  a. Lift the patient back up and into bed
  b. Immediately call for the nurse
  c. Document that the patient "sat on the floor"
  d. Ask another nurse aide to assist getting with the patient back up

34. Which food is appropriate for a patient on a full-liquid diet?

  a. Scrambled eggs
  b. Cooked vegetables
  c. Custard
  d. Cottage cheese

35. If a patient has been alone in a double room but is to receive a roommate with a new admission, what should the nurse aide do?

  a. Advise the patient before bringing the new patient into the room
  b. Wait until after the new patient is in the room to explain
  c. Ask the patient if he or she wants a roommate
  d. Remind the patient that he or she has no control over roommates

36. At what point should colostomy or ileostomy bag be emptied?
   a. At the end of each shift
   b. Every 4 hours
   c. When it is completely full
   d. When it is one-third to one-half full

37. A patient who has been newly admitted to a long-term-care facility has brought a number of mementos—pictures, knickknacks, figurines, books—into her single room. How should the nurse aide respond?
   a. Tell the patient to send them home
   b. Label them with the patient's name
   c. Warn the patient that they might get lost or stolen
   d. Ask the patient if so many things are really necessary

38. If using a position change alarm in a patient's wheelchair (WC), which of the following is true?
   a. The alarm should be tested before the patient is left unattended.
   b. The alarm should be at least 4 feet from the patient's ears.
   c. The alarm should be within easy reach of the patient.
   d. The alarm should be near the patient's head to alert the patient to danger.

39. A newly trained nurse aide has been delegated a task that the nurse aide does not feel adequately prepared to do. What should the nurse aide do?
   a. Ask another nurse aide for assistance
   b. Ask a supervisor for assistance
   c. Make an excuse for why the nurse aide cannot do the task
   d. Explain the concerns to the delegating nurse

40. If a patient has a visitor who is unkempt and appears homeless, how should the nurse aide respond?
   a. Discreetly watch the visitor
   b. Offer the visitor toiletries
   c. Treat the visitor with respect
   d. Ask why the patient has a homeless visitor

41. Which of the following is a boundary violation?
   a. The nurse aide accepts a box of candy to be shared by the entire staff.
   b. The nurse aide helps a patient write a personal letter.
   c. The nurse aide listens while the patient tells the nurse aide about family problems.
   d. The nurse aide accepts a plant that the patient gives the nurse aide on discharge.

42. If moving a patient to the side of the bed in preparation for turning, which part of the patient should the nurse aide move first?
   a. Legs and feet
   b. Head and upper body
   c. Lower part of the body (abdomen and buttocks)
   d. Arm and leg on the side toward the move

43. At what point may an alcohol-based hand sanitizer be used for hand hygiene?

    a. When hands are soiled with body fluids

    b. After exposure to a patient with infectious diarrhea

    c. After contact with a patient's intact skin

    d. After using the restroom

44. What is the normal range for the pulse rate of a 20-year-old patient?

    a. 60–100

    b. 50–90

    c. 70–80

    d. 50–70

45. If sterilizing items, such as bandage scissors, in the home environment, the items should be boiled (at sea level) for how long?

    a. 5 minutes

    b. 10 minutes

    c. 15 minutes

    d. 20 minutes

46. A patient with a head injury is to remain in the semi-Fowler's position. To what angle should the head of the bed (HOB) be raised?

    a. 30°

    b. 45°

    c. 60°

    d. 90°

47. Before cutting a patient's fingernails, how long should the nurse aide soak the patient's fingers?

    a. 1–2 minutes

    b. 2–5 minutes

    c. 5–10 minutes

    d. 10–15 minutes

48. If an older adult needs mouth care, what is the best tool?

    a. A medium-to-hard bristle toothbrush

    b. A sponge swab

    c. Mouthwash

    d. A soft-bristle toothbrush

49. If a patient's skin rubs against the sheets when the patient is repositioned in bed, this is referred to as which of the following?

    a. Shearing

    b. Bruising

    c. Friction

    d. Tearing

50. For a 2-year-old child, how far should a rectal thermometer be inserted?

   a. 0.5 inches
   b. 1 inch
   c. 1.5 inches
   d. 2 inches

51. If a knee is in a flexed position, that means the knee is which of the following?

   a. Bent
   b. Straight
   c. Swollen
   d. Twisted

52. A patient's Foley catheter urinary drainage bag is full. How should the nurse aide empty the bag?

   a. Replace the tubing and drainage bag with a new set
   b. Disconnect the tubing, plug the catheter, and take the drainage bag to the bathroom to measure the urine
   c. Open the clamp on the drainage spout and empty the urine into a bedpan before measuring
   d. Open the clamp on the drainage spout and empty the urine directly into a measuring cup

53. When carrying out range-of-motion (ROM) exercises and the nurse aide meets resistance, what should the nurse aide do?

   a. Continue with the exercises but more gently
   b. Stop and notify the nurse
   c. Push the joint past the resistance
   d. Continue to the point of pain

54. If a patient requires a jacket restraint while in a WC, what must be done?

   a. Position the straps at a 45° angle between the seat and the sides
   b. Be sure the jacket opening is in the front
   c. Place a pillow behind the patient's back
   d. Be sure that the jacket is loose enough that the patient can move freely

55. If the nurse tells the nurse aide that a patient can have pain medication "prn," what does this mean?

   a. Before meals
   b. After meals
   c. As needed
   d. Every 4 hours

56. An 8-year-old child is alone in a hospital room and is frightened. How should the nurse aide respond?

   a. Give the child a toy
   b. Turn on the TV
   c. Sit and talk to the child
   d. Tell the nurse

57. Which of the following is true for airborne precautions?

    a. The patient should be placed in a standard single room

    b. Gowns and gloves should be worn for all patient contact

    c. The patient's door should be propped open for easy access

    d. An approved respirator (such as N95) must be worn when caring for the patient

58. What is the difference between an open and a closed bed?

    a. An open bed does not have top linens.

    b. An open bed has the top linens fan-folded to one side of the bed.

    c. An open bed has the top linens covering the bottom linens.

    d. An open bed has the top linens fan-folded to the foot.

59. A native healer is visiting a patient and is in the middle of a healing ritual when the nurse aide enters the room to feed the patient. How should the nurse aide respond?

    a. Leave the room and close the door or curtains

    b. Tell the healer that the patient needs to eat

    c. Interrupt and ask when the healer will be finished

    d. Ask if the healer has permission to conduct a ritual

60. Which of the following is the best approach if raising a patient's head and shoulders to adjust the patient's pillows?

    a. Pull the patient upright by the arm

    b. Push the patient's head and back from behind

    c. Lock arms with the patient

    d. Get help from another staff member

61. If a patient who is dying is increasingly rude toward family members who are in good health, which stage of dying (Kübler-Ross) is the patient exhibiting?

    a. Denial

    b. Anger

    c. Bargaining

    d. Depression

62. A patient weighs 800 pounds and does not fit into a regular bed, so a bariatric bed is being brought to accommodate the patient. What should the nurse aide tell the patient?

    a. "You are too heavy for a regular bed, so we're getting a bed that can handle your weight."

    b. "You need a special bariatric bed for patients who are overweight."

    c. "We're getting you a bigger bed."

    d. "We're getting a bed that will be more comfortable for you."

63. If the nurse aide is giving a cleansing enema to a bed patient, how high above the anus should the enema bag generally be hung?

    a. 6 inches

    b. 8 inches

    c. 12 inches

    d. 18 inches

64. If a patient repeatedly coughs while the nurse aide is feeding the patient, what should the nurse aide do?
 a. Stop the feeding and tell the nurse
 b. Feed the patient more slowly
 c. Offer liquid after every bite
 d. Give the patient smaller spoonfuls of food

65. When entering the room of a patient who is completely blind, which of the following should the nurse aide do?
 a. Clap their hands to alert the patient.
 b. Stop and state their name, title, and purpose.
 c. Touch the patient gently to alert the patient to their presence.
 d. Say the patient's name to alert the patient to their presence.

66. Following surgery, how frequently should a patient be assisted to carry out deep breathing and coughing exercises?
 a. Every 4–6 hours
 b. Every 2–4 hours
 c. Every 1–2 hours
 d. Every 30–60 minutes

67. When a patient is admitted to a facility, what information may the nurse aide be expected to gather from the patient?
 a. Height and weight
 b. Reason for admission
 c. Mental status
 d. List of medications

68. When identifying a patient, which of the following may serve as two appropriate identifiers?
 a. Room and bed number
 b. First and last name
 c. Name and birthdate
 d. Telephone number and street address

69. When collecting a urine specimen from a patient who is ambulatory, the nurse aide should do which of the following?
 a. Give the patient a cup to urinate into
 b. Place a specimen pan into the toilet
 c. Ask the patient to urinate into a bedpan in bed
 d. Place a bedpan on top of the toilet

70. If a patient is using an incentive spirometer, the nurse aide should ask the patient to seal the lips around the mouthpiece and then do what?
 a. Inhale as much as possible and hold their breath for 2–3 seconds
 b. Exhale as much as possible and hold their breath for 2–3 seconds
 c. Inhale as rapidly as possible and hold their breath for 2–3 seconds
 d. Exhale as rapidly as possible and hold their breath for 2–3 seconds

Answer Key and Explanations for Test #3

1. B: If a patient is to use crutches because of no weight bearing on one leg, the type of gait that the patient will use is three-point. All other gaits require at least partial weight bearing on both legs. With the three-point gait, all weight is on one foot. The patient stands on one foot supported by the crutches, moves both crutches forward at the same time, and then swings the foot to the new position at or past the crutches, depending on the patient's strength and mobility.

2. D: If a home health aide is caring for a patient and inadvertently receives a needlestick injury with a used insulin syringe, the nurse aide should report the exposure to the home health agency immediately. Although not required by law to have human immunodeficiency virus or hepatitis B testing, the agency is responsible for paying for testing if the nurse aide chooses to have it. Blood can also be drawn and held for 90 days in case the nurse aide wants testing at a later time.

3. B: Before obtaining a sputum specimen, the nurse aide should ask the patient to rinse the mouth with water in case there is any debris in the patient's mouth. If possible, place the patient in a sitting position and ask the patient to hold the container, take two or three deep breaths, and then cough directly into the specimen container. Usually, 1–2 teaspoons of sputum are needed for testing. The nurse should specify if a larger specimen is needed.

4. C: If a patient has been incontinent of urine in bed, an appropriate response is, "Let me help you get clean right away." The nurse aide should not try to embarrass the patient or indicate that the incident should have been avoided, but should handle the incident matter-of-factly. When finished, the nurse aide should make sure that the patient's call bell is within reach. If this is a new problem, the nurse aide should notify the nurse because the patient may have an infection or other problem.

5. A: Standard precautions include wearing PPE when in contact with blood or body fluids or nonintact skin, although PPE is not needed for indirect contact or contact with intact skin. PPE includes gloves and gowns. If there is a risk of splashing body fluids, then masks, goggles, and/or face shields should also be used. PPE should not be reused, even for the same patient, except in emergency situations when fresh PPE is not available. Patients should be at least 3 feet apart with a curtain closed between them.

6. D: Pressure injuries most often occur over bony prominences where the tissue is caught between the bone internally and compression externally. Pressure injury stages are listed below:

- Suspected deep-tissue injury: Skin discolored, intact or blood blister.
- Stage I: Intact skin with a nonblanching reddened area.
- Stage II: Abrasion or blistered area without slough but with partial-thickness skin loss.
- Stage III: Deep ulcer with exposed subcutaneous tissue. Tunneling or undermining may be evident with or without slough.
- Stage IV: Deep ulcer, full thickness, with necrosis into muscle, bone, tendons, and/or joints.
- Unstageable: Eschar and/or slough prevents staging prior to debridement.

7. B: If a patient is to drink 1 liter of water as prep for a colonoscopy, this is equal to 1,000 mL. A liter is slightly larger than a quart, which is equal to 32 ounces (960 mL). The metric system is used in medicine because it is more precise and can better measure very small quantities than the

158

imperial system. Patients who are on intake and output measurement must have both calculated in milliliters (mL) rather than ounces, so the ounces must be converted to mL:

- 1 ounce = 30 mL
- 4 ounces = 120 mL
- 8 ounces (1 cup) = 240 mL

8. C: School-age children (6–12 years old) need to sleep approximately 9–12 hours per day. Sleep needs based on age are listed as follows:

Neonate (0–3 months)	14–17 hours
Infant (4–12 months)	12–16 hours
Toddler (1–2 years)	11–14 hours
Preschool (3–5 years)	10–13 hours
School-age (6–12 years)	9–12 hours
Adolescent (13–18 years)	8–10 hours
Adult (18+)	7–9 hours

9. B: Although intravenous medications take effect immediately, subcutaneous injections usually within about 5 minutes, and intramuscular injections within 5–10 minutes, oral medications usually take 20–30 minutes before they are effective, so the nurse aide should wait that long to ensure that the patient is comfortable before getting the patient up to sit in the chair. The times are only approximate because individual response may vary, so the nurse aide should be guided by the patient.

10. A: If changing a front-opening gown while the patient is in bed, the first step is to undo the fasteners (buttons, zippers, ties) and then to slide the gown off of the shoulders and off of an arm (if one is weak, use the stronger arm). Then, raise the patient and gather the gown toward the opposite side. Lower the patient and then remove the gown from the other arm and gather the gown under the patient. Turn the patient to remove the gathered gown.

11. C: A cleansing enema (500–1,000 mL) should be administered over 10–15 minutes, so the flow should be slow. If administered too rapidly, the patient may experience cramps and some of the enema solution may quickly run back out. Cleansing enemas include:

- Tap water enemas: No more than one enema should be given because it may cause fluid imbalance if some fluid is absorbed.
- Normal saline enemas (2 tablespoons salt to 500–1,000 mL water): May cause fluid retention because of sodium absorption.
- Soapsuds enemas (3–5 mL castile soap per 500–1,000 mL water): May be irritating to intestinal tissues, especially if too much soap is used.

12. A: If a patient wears disposable incontinence briefs for urinary and fecal incontinence, the nurse aide should provide perineal care after each episode of incontinence. Patients who are incontinent should be checked on a regular schedule, such as every 2–3 hours, to determine if they need to be changed. A skin barrier, such as zinc oxide cream, may be used to protect the skin, and the skin should be examined carefully for signs of irritation with each perineal care session.

13. D: Before bedtime, a gentle back massage may help a patient to relax so that the patient can sleep better. Tea contains caffeine, which is a stimulant, and should be avoided. A bath or hot shower should be taken at least 1 hour before bed, and physical exercise, which may have a stimulating rather than a relaxing effect, should be avoided before bedtime. Other types of relaxation exercises, such as deep breathing and visualization, may also help the patient to relax.

14. B: If a nurse aide notices that a patient assigned to another nurse aide is trying to drink water but is having difficulty raising the glass, the nurse aide should offer to assist the patient. A patient's immediate needs should always be taken care of by whatever staff member is available regardless of who is assigned to the patient. Although a nurse aide may be assigned to patients for specific aspects of care, such as bathing and taking routine vital signs, they still have a duty of care to all patients on the unit in need of assistance.

15. A: The nurse aide may carry out a delegated task if it is within the nurse aide's range of functions, and this range may vary somewhat from one state and one facility to another, so it's important that the nurse aide understand the types of tasks that can be delegated to the nurse aide. Even if a nurse delegates a task that the nurse aide knows how to do, such as cutting toenails, the nurse aide can only do it if it is a permitted task.

16. C: If the healthcare organization uses electronic health records to document patient care, the nurse aide should guard the personal username and password from everyone else and should never share them with others. The nurse aide should also never log in for others who have forgotten their username or passwords because any action others carry out will be traced back to that nurse aide. The nurse aide should never write the username and password down on a card and carry it in a pocket because it may get lost.

17. D: The electronic communication to a friend that is acceptable under the Health Insurance Portability and Accountability Act of 1996 for a nurse aide working in home health care is "My last patient of the day lives near Pizza Palace, so I'll meet you there." The nurse aide should not divulge any personally identifying information about a patient, such as the patient's name or address and should never take or post personal pictures of a patient on social media. In most cases, the nurse aide should avoid any postings that refer to work or patients, even without identifying information.

18. A: To use proper body mechanics, the nurse aide should avoid stretching overhead more than 20 inches to reach items. The nurse aide should use a step stool or a grip tool. Preventive body mechanics include the following:

- Avoid bending at the waist to lift or reach for items. Stoop with bent knees.
- Avoid stretching overhead to reach for items out of reach (more than 20 inches). Use a step stool or grip tool with an extension.
- Avoid pulling—push, roll, or slide instead.
- Avoid lifting—pull, push, roll, or slide instead.
- Avoid reaching, bending, or twisting to lift.
- Avoid lifting. Use lift devices or get help.
- Avoid prolonged periods of repetitive activity.

19. B: Because the skin of older adults tends to be more friable and less well-lubricated than that of younger adults, unless the patient is soiled, the patient needs to have a complete bath only twice weekly. Older adults also perspire less. Soap is drying to the skin, so after an older adult bathes, lotion or cream should be applied to the skin. Between baths, the older patient may have a partial bath (face, underarms, perineal area, feet).

20. C: Before shaving a male patient's face with a safety razor, the nurse aide should first apply a warm moist cloth to his face to soften the beard for a few minutes. Then, the face is dried, and talcum powder may be applied if the patient wishes before using an electric shaver. Soap and water or shaving cream should be applied before shaving with a safety razor. Shaving should be done in the direction of hair growth with a safety razor but against the hair growth with an electric razor. Safety razors should never be used if a patient is on anticoagulants (blood thinners). Direct pressure should be applied to any nicks in the skin until the bleeding stops.

21. A: If using a shampoo cap to wash a patient's hair, the first step is to warm the cap (usually in a microwave), following the manufacturer's directions. Then, the nurse aide should check to make sure that the temperature is comfortable before applying the cap to the patient's head. The scalp is massaged through the cap for about 1–3 minutes, and then the cap is removed. The cleansing solution does not need to be rinsed from the hair. The hair may feel damp and need to be dried with a towel and then should be combed and brushed.

22. D: The role that the nurse aide serves as part of a team in the nursing process is reporting observations. Although these observations are often invaluable and help the nurse to develop a care plan and assess the patient's condition, the nurse's responsibility is to develop goals, assess patient progress, and assess patients' medical needs. The five steps of the nursing process are assessment, nursing diagnosis, planning, implementation, and evaluation.

23. B: If a patient with Alzheimer's disease insists on carrying a baby doll with her at all times and talks to the doll as though it is a real person, the nurse aide should ensure that the patient always has the doll. The doll obviously provides comfort to the patient and meets a need. Trying to orient the patient to the reality that the doll is not a real person is likely to only cause stress to the patient, and the nurse aide cannot accept the delusion without actively encouraging it.

24. A: A stand-pivot transfer is appropriate if the patient can assist with the transfer. The patient's legs must be strong enough to be able to bear some or all of the body weight, and the patient must be able to follow simple directions. If transferring from bed to wheelchair (WC), the WC should be next to the patient at a 90º angle. The foot closest to the WC is moved forward, and the other foot is moved back. The patient may stand with a walker or with the help of the nurse aide who wraps his or her arms around the patient's torso under the arms. The patient stands and then is assisted to turn and sit into the WC.

25. C: If a patient's son asks the nurse aide why the patient is no longer receiving physical therapy, the nurse aide should refer the son to the nurse for further information. The nurse aide should also offer to take the question to the nurse and ask the nurse to come to speak to the son. Discussing medical treatments and the reasons why a patient may or may not be receiving them is within the scope of practice of the nurse but is not in the range of functions of the nurse aide.

26. D: Because the pulse oximeter fits on a finger, it can easily come loose, so if a patient's oxygen saturation per pulse oximeter has consistently been 95–97% but suddenly drops to 78% and the patient shows no signs of respiratory distress, the nurse aide should immediately reposition the pulse oximeter. If there is no improvement, then the nurse aide should report the finding to the nurse. If the patient is not in distress but the oxygen saturation level remains low, the problem may be with the pulse oximeter.

27. B: Although all of these observations should be reported to the nurse, the one that should be reported immediately is a sudden loss of vision in one eye because this is an abnormal finding that requires assessment by the nurse, who will then determine if the physician should be notified. Any observation that may threaten the health or well-being of a patient should be reported immediately as well as any observation about which the nurse aide is uncertain.

28. A: Bedbound patients should be repositioned at least every 1–2 hours. In some cases, patients may be able to reposition themselves, but many patients need assistance or reminders. The nurse should indicate the necessary frequency as part of the patient's care plan. When repositioning a patient, the nurse aide should always examine the patient's skin and report any signs of redness that might indicate an increased risk for a pressure sore.

29. C: The directional term that is used to describe the body part that is closest to the center or to the point of attachment is proximal. Thus, the proximal part of the arm is the upper arm and the distal part is the lower arm. Medial is toward the midline, whereas lateral is away from the midline and to the side. Anterior is toward the front, and posterior is toward the back. Superior is toward the head or above, and inferior is toward the feet or below. When describing an area of the patient's body, the description should be patient-oriented, using phrases such as "patient's left" and "patient's right" to ensure accurate interpretation.

30. B: When reporting to a nurse about an older adult patient—or any adult patient—the nurse aide should address the patient by title and last name ("Miss Brown"). The same is true when directly addressing the patient. Terms of endearment ("Honey" or "Sweetie") are not appropriate. If a patient requests that the nurse aide use the patient's first name, then this is appropriate when directly addressing the patient but not when reporting on the patient. No patient should be referred to by room and bed number alone.

31. D: If a procedure needs to be done "stat," this means immediately. Most often, stat orders are given with regard to medications or treatments. For example, if a patient is in severe pain, an analgesia may be ordered "stat and q 6 hours prn," meaning immediately and then every 6 hours as needed. In some cases, a nurse may request that something, such as assisting a patient to the bathroom, be done "stat" to stress the importance of doing the task right away.

32. A: If a long-term-care patient does not want to participate in group activities, the nurse aide should ask what the patient would prefer to do. Patients have the right to refuse not only treatments but also activities and should not be coerced into participation or asked to explain themselves. However, it is appropriate to determine what the patient's interests are. Opportunities for participation should still be offered to the patient.

33. B: If a patient slips onto the floor during a transfer but appears uninjured, the nurse aide should remain with the patient and immediately use the call bell to call for the nurse to report what happened. The nurse aide should not attempt to move the patient until after the nurse has examined the patient for potential injuries. Any time a patient falls to the floor, an incident report must be filled out describing what happened, when and how it happened, and who witnessed the incident.

34. C: The food that is appropriate for a patient on a full-liquid diet is custard. Full-liquid diets include all foods that are essentially liquid at room temperature or if heated, including clear liquids (water, apple juice, and cranberry juice), as well as other juices (orange juice, pineapple juice, and tomato juice) and milk products, including eggnog, puddings, and ice cream. Soups may be strained and the broth may be eaten. A full-liquid diet does not include pureed foods or cooked vegetables.

35. A: If a patient has been alone in a double room but is to receive a roommate with a new admission, the nurse aide should advise the patient before bringing the new patient into the room. Even though the patient has no control over who else is assigned to the room, it is courteous to advise the patient and to make sure that the patient's things are not in the other person's space. The nurse aide may introduce the patients but should provide no information about the new patient's condition.

36. D: A colostomy or ileostomy bag should be emptied when it is one-third to one-half full in order to prevent leakage and odor as well as bulging of the bag under the patient's clothing. If the appliance is leaking under the seal, the entire appliance should be changed. If the bag is drainable, it can be drained into the toilet or into a bedpan. In some cases, the bag itself is removed and changed, but the base disk applied to the skin remains in place.

37. B: If a patient who has been newly admitted to a long-term-care facility has brought a number of mementos—pictures, knickknacks, figurines, books—into her single room, the nurse aide should label them with the patient's name in case they get misplaced. Within the limits set at each facility, patients have the right to bring personal items of their choice. Being surrounded by personal belongings can be comforting to patients and help them cope with the change to a new environment.

38. A: If using a position change alarm in a patient's WC, the alarm should be tested before the patient is left unattended to ensure that it is working properly. The alarm should be at least 2 feet from the patient's ears, especially if it is quite loud, and it should be out of reach of the patient. Position change alarms should not be so sensitive that the slightest move sets off the alarm because this is stressful to the patient and over time and repeated false alarms tend to be ignored by staff.

39. D: If a newly trained nurse aide has been delegated a task that the nurse aide does not feel adequately prepared to do, the nurse aide should explain the concerns to the delegating nurse. Because it's the nurse's responsibility to supervise the nurse aide, the nurse should be willing to assist and help the nurse aide to complete the task. With experience, the nurse aide will increase in confidence and skills.

40. C: If a patient has a visitor who is unkempt and appears homeless, the nurse aide should treat the visitor with respect, the same as any other visitor. It's not appropriate for staff members to police a patient's visitors without cause based on stereotypes, and one can't always make accurate assumptions based on appearances. A person, for example, may be unkempt after working as a laborer all day or may be homeless because of the loss of a job or due to sickness.

41. D: It is a boundary violation to accept a personal gift, such as a plant, from a patient even though the gift may seem quite insignificant. The nurse aide should thank the patient and explain the facility's policy against accepting any gifts. At most facilities, it is acceptable to accept a gift of candy if it is intended for the entire staff and not just an individual, but each facility should have clear policies in place about the appropriateness of accepting such gifts.

42. B: If moving a patient to the side of the bed in preparation for turning, the nurse aide should first move the head and upper body and then the lower part of the body (abdomen and buttocks). The legs and feet are moved last. The patient may be moved by placing one arm under the patient's body and one arm over, or the patient can be moved with a turning sheet or a draw sheet with the help of another person.

43. C: An alcohol-based hand sanitizer may be used for hand hygiene after contact with a patient's intact skin and before direct contact with a patient. An alcohol-based hand sanitizer may also be used after contact with body fluids (other than blood) if there is no visible soiling, but if any soiling is present at all, the hands should be washed thoroughly with soap and water. The hands should also be washed with soap and water before and after using the restroom or eating and after exposure to a patient with infectious diarrhea.

44. A: The normal range for the pulse rate of a patient age 20 is 60–100. Some people may have a slower pulse rate (45–60), especially people who are very athletic and women who are small in stature. Crying, stress, fear, and pain can all increase the pulse rate.

Age	Normal pulse/minute
0–1 year	80–190
2 years	80–160
6 years	75–120
10 years	70–110
12 through adulthood	60–100

45. B: If sterilizing items, such as bandage scissors, in the home environment, the items should be boiled (at sea level) for 10 minutes. For each 1,000 feet above sea level, the boiling time should be extended by 1 minutes. So, if a patient is located in an area that is 4,000 feet above sea level, then the items should be boiled for 14 minutes (10 minutes plus 4 minutes). Only the actual boiling time is counted, not the time it takes to reach a boil. Therefore, some guidelines specify that tools should be boiled for 20 minutes to be on the safe side.

46. A: If a patient with a head injury is to remain in the semi-Fowler's position, the HOB should be raised to 30º. The positions are listed as follows:

- Fowler's: HOB 45–60º.
- Semi-Fowler's: HOB 30º.
- High Fowler's: HOB 60–90º.
- Supine: Flat on the back.
- Prone: Abdomen down.
- Lateral: Right or left side.
- Sims': Left side with the right knee flexed and the left arm and leg behind the patient.

47. C: Before cutting a patient's fingernails, the nurse aide should soak the patient's fingers for 5–10 minutes to dislodge any debris under the nails and to soften the nails so they are easier to cut. The nails should be cleaned with an orangewood stick and the cuticles should be pushed back with the orangewood stick or with a cloth. The nails should be cut straight across with clippers, and then the edges are rounded with a nail file or emery board. The nurse aide should check each finger to ensure that the nails are smooth to avoid the nails catching and tearing.

48. D: If an older adult needs mouth care, the best tool is a soft-bristle toothbrush. The teeth should be brushed gently but thoroughly with the brush held at a 45º angle to the teeth. The nurse aide may also floss the teeth before or after brushing using a flosser or an 18-inch piece of floss. Mouthwash may be added to the water to rinse the mouth, but mouthwash cannot take the place of brushing. Flossing generally starts in the upper right and moves around to the upper left followed by flossing of the bottom teeth.

49. C: If a patient's skin rubs against the sheets when the patient is repositioned in bed, this is referred to as friction. Friction may also occur when one body part rubs against another. To prevent friction when moving a patient, the nurse aide should use friction-reducing devices, such as a lift sheet, and should get help to move patients. Friction irritates the outer layers of the skin and makes the tissue more susceptible to pressure injuries, especially if shearing is also involved.

50. B: For a 2-year-old child, a rectal thermometer should be inserted 1 inch. Rectal temperature measurements are typically used only for infants and children younger than 3 years old. A digital thermometer is the best choice for a rectal thermometer because it registers the temperature quickly. An infant can be placed on the abdomen or on the back and legs lifted to expose the anus. A young child may be placed in the Sims' position. The thermometer should be lubricated and inserted one-half inch for infants younger than 6 months old and one inch for older infants and young children. The normal range for a rectal temperature is 37.0–38.1 ℃.

51. A: If the knee is in a flexed position, the knee is bent. Flexed is the opposite of extended, which is straight. If a joint is hyperextended, it is excessively straightened, usually resulting in injury to the joint. Internal rotation is turning a joint inward, and external rotation is turning a joint outward. Dorsiflexion is bending the foot upward at the ankle, and plantar flexion is bending the foot downward at the ankle. Pronation is turning a joint downward, and supination is turning a joint upward.

52. D: If a patient's Foley catheter urinary drainage bag is full, to empty the bag, the nurse aide should open the clamp on the drainage spout and empty the urine directly into a measuring cup, taking care not to touch the spout to the container. A bedpan is considered dirty and should not be used to collect urine. Foley drainage bags are typically emptied when they are full or at least at the end of each 8-hour period.

53. B: If, when carrying out ROM exercises and the nurse aide meets resistance, the nurse aide should stop and notify the nurse. The nurse should examine the joint to assess the possible causes for the resistance and should determine whether ROM exercises should continue or whether the joint should be rested. Continuing with ROM exercises when resistance is encountered could result in pain and discomfort to the patient and injury to the joint.

54. A: If a patient requires a jacket restraint while in a WC, position the straps at a 45º angle between the seat and the sides. The jacket restraint opens in the back so that the patient cannot easily remove it. No pillow or support should be placed behind the patient's back because the patient should be positioned with the back against the back of the WC and sitting upright. The jacket should be applied so that it is snug but still comfortable.

55. C: If the nurse tells the nurse aide that a patient can have pain medication "prn," this means "as needed," although there are usually still restrictions, such as "prn q 4 h," which means "as needed every 4 hours." The nurse aide often has close contact with patients and may be the first to notice that a patient is in pain and should always report this to the nurse so that the patient can receive pain medication to relieve any discomfort.

56. C: If an 8-year-old child is alone in a hospital room and is frightened, the nurse aide should sit and talk to the child. Children are especially frightened of the unknown, so the nurse aide can talk about what the child should expect—such as when mealtimes are, when the child will receive treatments, when family/caregivers will return. The nurse aide may talk about the child's interests and favorite activities. If toys or TV are available, the nurse aide may offer them to the child as well.

57. D: For airborne precautions, an approved respirator (such as N95) must be worn when caring for the patient. The N95 should be fitted to the individual. Airborne diseases (COVID-19, measles, tuberculosis, and chicken pox) are spread through the respiratory tract. Patients should be placed in a negative-pressure room that is vented to the outside to reduce the risk of transmission to others. If possible, the patient should be placed in a single-occupancy room.

58. D: The difference between an open and a closed bed is that the open bed has the top linens fan-folded to the foot of the bed to make it easy for a patient to get into the bed whereas the closed bed has the top linens in place and covering the bottom linens. The surgical bed has the linens fan-folded to one side. After making the open bed, the nurse places the towels, bath blanket, and gown or pajamas in the bedside stand so they are in place when the patient arrives.

59. A: If a native healer is visiting a patient and is in the middle of a healing ritual when the nurse aide enters the room to feed the patient, the nurse aide should leave the room and close the door or curtains. Although the patient's food may need to be reheated, the healing ritual is likely more important to the patient than eating on time. Patients have the right to observe their own spiritual, cultural, and religious practices while hospitalized.

60. C: If raising a patient's head and shoulders to adjust the patient's pillow, the best approach is to lock arms with the patient. Facing the patient, the nurse aide places the near arm under the patient's axilla to grasp the shoulder while the patient does the same, grasping the nurse aide's shoulder. The nurse aide then turns and places the far arm under the patient's neck and shoulders. Then the nurse aide raises the patient and uses the far arm to adjust the pillow before lowering the patient again.

61. B: If a patient who is dying is increasingly rude toward family members who are in good health, the stage of dying that the patient is exhibiting is anger. The stages of dying (Kübler-Ross) include

- Stage 1—Denial: Disbelieving, confused, stunned, detached, repeating questions.
- Stage 2—Anger: Directed inward (self-blame) or outward.
- Stage 3—Bargaining: If–then thinking (If I go to church, then I will heal). Trying to find a different outcome.
- Stage 4—Depression: Sad, withdrawn, tearful, crying but beginning to accept the loss.
- Stage 5—Acceptance: Resolution and acceptance.

Patients may not go through every stage, and the stages are not always sequential. Some patients become fixed at one stage, such as anger or denial.

62. D: If a patient weighs 800 pounds and does not fit into a regular bed and a bariatric bed is being brought to accommodate the patient, the nurse aide should tell the patient, "We're getting a bed that will be more comfortable for you." Patients who are obese are well aware of this fact, so the nurse aide should avoid saying anything that may embarrass the patient or focus on the patient's weight rather than on the patient's needs.

63. C: If the nurse aide is giving a cleansing enema to a bed patient, the enema bag should generally be hung 12 inches above the anus to allow a free flow of fluid by gravity but without excess pressure (which increases as the height increases). The enema solution should be lukewarm, and the nurse aide should check the temperature before administration. The patient is placed in the left Sims' position for the enema. The lubricated tube should be inserted 2–4 inches inside an adult's rectum.

64. A: If a patient repeatedly coughs while the nurse aide is feeding the patient, the nurse aide should stop feeding the patient and tell the nurse so that the nurse can examine the patient to determine if the patient is aspirating, which means that some of the food and/or fluid is entering the lungs instead of the stomach. Other signs of aspiration may include pain when swallowing, difficulty initiating a swallow, wheezing, excessive saliva, and chest discomfort.

65. B: When entering the room of a patient who is completely blind, the nurse aide should stop and state his or her name, title, and purpose: "Mrs. Brown, this is Sally Smith, your nurse aide. I'm here to help you take your shower." If the patient is in a single room, the nurse aide should stop at the door. If the patient is in a double room, the nurse aide should stop at a distance from the bed.

People who are blind can often sense or hear the presence of another person and may be startled if the nurse aide approaches too closely before speaking.

66. C: Following surgery, a patient should be assisted to carry out deep breathing and coughing exercises every 1–2 hours during waking hours in order to prevent pneumonia and atelectasis (collapse of part of the lung because of underventilation). The procedure for deep breathing and coughing is as follows:

- For abdominal or chest incisions, support the surgical site with the hands or a pillow before beginning the exercise.
- Take two or three deep breaths and exhale.
- Take a deep breath and hold for 2–3 seconds.
- Cough two times.

67. A: When a patient is admitted to a facility, the information that the nurse aide may be expected to gather includes the patient's height and weight. The admission interview and assessment should be carried out by a nurse, although the nurse may delegate some tasks, such as recording the patient's height and weight and vital signs and making a clothing and belongings list. The nurse aide also prepares the room before the patient's arrival.

68. C: When identifying a patient, two appropriate identifiers include the patient's name and birthdate. Most facilities require that the nurse aide check the patient's identification band as well. The nurse aide should ask the patient to provide information, "What is your name and birthdate?" rather than asking the patient to confirm information, "Is your name Molly Brown?" Patients who are confused or disoriented may not answer questions appropriately.

69. B: When collecting a urine specimen from a patient who is ambulatory, the nurse aide should place a specimen pan into the toilet, under the toilet seat. The nurse aide should be sure to advise the patient not to put the toilet paper into the specimen, which is collected at the front of the container. The urine specimen should be poured into a urine specimen container, which must be properly labeled as a biohazard. The nurse aide should try to collect about 4 ounces (120 mL) of urine for the specimen.

70. A: If a patient is using an incentive spirometer, the nurse aide should ask the patient to seal the lips around the mouthpiece, inhale as much as possible, and hold the breath for 2–3 seconds. The purpose of the incentive spirometer is to help to expand the lungs and prevent atelectasis. The patient should inhale at a slow, steady rate, trying to raise the device's piston to the target level.

How to Overcome Test Anxiety

Just the thought of taking a test is enough to make most people a little nervous. A test is an important event that can have a long-term impact on your future, so it's important to take it seriously and it's natural to feel anxious about performing well. But just because anxiety is normal, that doesn't mean that it's helpful in test taking, or that you should simply accept it as part of your life. Anxiety can have a variety of effects. These effects can be mild, like making you feel slightly nervous, or severe, like blocking your ability to focus or remember even a simple detail.

If you experience test anxiety—whether severe or mild—it's important to know how to beat it. To discover this, first you need to understand what causes test anxiety.

Causes of Test Anxiety

While we often think of anxiety as an uncontrollable emotional state, it can actually be caused by simple, practical things. One of the most common causes of test anxiety is that a person does not feel adequately prepared for their test. This feeling can be the result of many different issues such as poor study habits or lack of organization, but the most common culprit is time management. Starting to study too late, failing to organize your study time to cover all of the material, or being distracted while you study will mean that you're not well prepared for the test. This may lead to cramming the night before, which will cause you to be physically and mentally exhausted for the test. Poor time management also contributes to feelings of stress, fear, and hopelessness as you realize you are not well prepared but don't know what to do about it.

Other times, test anxiety is not related to your preparation for the test but comes from unresolved fear. This may be a past failure on a test, or poor performance on tests in general. It may come from comparing yourself to others who seem to be performing better or from the stress of living up to expectations. Anxiety may be driven by fears of the future—how failure on this test would affect your educational and career goals. These fears are often completely irrational, but they can still negatively impact your test performance.

> **Review Video: 3 Reasons You Have Test Anxiety**
> Visit mometrix.com/academy and enter code: 428468

Elements of Test Anxiety

As mentioned earlier, test anxiety is considered to be an emotional state, but it has physical and mental components as well. Sometimes you may not even realize that you are suffering from test anxiety until you notice the physical symptoms. These can include trembling hands, rapid heartbeat, sweating, nausea, and tense muscles. Extreme anxiety may lead to fainting or vomiting. Obviously, any of these symptoms can have a negative impact on testing. It is important to recognize them as soon as they begin to occur so that you can address the problem before it damages your performance.

> **Review Video: 3 Ways to Tell You Have Test Anxiety**
> Visit mometrix.com/academy and enter code: 927847

The mental components of test anxiety include trouble focusing and inability to remember learned information. During a test, your mind is on high alert, which can help you recall information and stay focused for an extended period of time. However, anxiety interferes with your mind's natural processes, causing you to blank out, even on the questions you know well. The strain of testing during anxiety makes it difficult to stay focused, especially on a test that may take several hours. Extreme anxiety can take a huge mental toll, making it difficult not only to recall test information but even to understand the test questions or pull your thoughts together.

> **Review Video: How Test Anxiety Affects Memory**
> Visit mometrix.com/academy and enter code: 609003

Effects of Test Anxiety

Test anxiety is like a disease—if left untreated, it will get progressively worse. Anxiety leads to poor performance, and this reinforces the feelings of fear and failure, which in turn lead to poor performances on subsequent tests. It can grow from a mild nervousness to a crippling condition. If allowed to progress, test anxiety can have a big impact on your schooling, and consequently on your future.

Test anxiety can spread to other parts of your life. Anxiety on tests can become anxiety in any stressful situation, and blanking on a test can turn into panicking in a job situation. But fortunately, you don't have to let anxiety rule your testing and determine your grades. There are a number of relatively simple steps you can take to move past anxiety and function normally on a test and in the rest of life.

> **Review Video: How Test Anxiety Impacts Your Grades**
> Visit mometrix.com/academy and enter code: 939819

Physical Steps for Beating Test Anxiety

While test anxiety is a serious problem, the good news is that it can be overcome. It doesn't have to control your ability to think and remember information. While it may take time, you can begin taking steps today to beat anxiety.

Just as your first hint that you may be struggling with anxiety comes from the physical symptoms, the first step to treating it is also physical. Rest is crucial for having a clear, strong mind. If you are tired, it is much easier to give in to anxiety. But if you establish good sleep habits, your body and mind will be ready to perform optimally, without the strain of exhaustion. Additionally, sleeping well helps you to retain information better, so you're more likely to recall the answers when you see the test questions.

Getting good sleep means more than going to bed on time. It's important to allow your brain time to relax. Take study breaks from time to time so it doesn't get overworked, and don't study right before bed. Take time to rest your mind before trying to rest your body, or you may find it difficult to fall asleep.

> **Review Video: <u>The Importance of Sleep for Your Brain</u>**
> Visit mometrix.com/academy and enter code: 319338

Along with sleep, other aspects of physical health are important in preparing for a test. Good nutrition is vital for good brain function. Sugary foods and drinks may give a burst of energy but this burst is followed by a crash, both physically and emotionally. Instead, fuel your body with protein and vitamin-rich foods.

Also, drink plenty of water. Dehydration can lead to headaches and exhaustion, especially if your brain is already under stress from the rigors of the test. Particularly if your test is a long one, drink water during the breaks. And if possible, take an energy-boosting snack to eat between sections.

> **Review Video: <u>How Diet Can Affect your Mood</u>**
> Visit mometrix.com/academy and enter code: 624317

Along with sleep and diet, a third important part of physical health is exercise. Maintaining a steady workout schedule is helpful, but even taking 5-minute study breaks to walk can help get your blood pumping faster and clear your head. Exercise also releases endorphins, which contribute to a positive feeling and can help combat test anxiety.

When you nurture your physical health, you are also contributing to your mental health. If your body is healthy, your mind is much more likely to be healthy as well. So take time to rest, nourish your body with healthy food and water, and get moving as much as possible. Taking these physical steps will make you stronger and more able to take the mental steps necessary to overcome test anxiety.

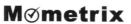

Mental Steps for Beating Test Anxiety

Working on the mental side of test anxiety can be more challenging, but as with the physical side, there are clear steps you can take to overcome it. As mentioned earlier, test anxiety often stems from lack of preparation, so the obvious solution is to prepare for the test. Effective studying may be the most important weapon you have for beating test anxiety, but you can and should employ several other mental tools to combat fear.

First, boost your confidence by reminding yourself of past success—tests or projects that you aced. If you're putting as much effort into preparing for this test as you did for those, there's no reason you should expect to fail here. Work hard to prepare; then trust your preparation.

Second, surround yourself with encouraging people. It can be helpful to find a study group, but be sure that the people you're around will encourage a positive attitude. If you spend time with others who are anxious or cynical, this will only contribute to your own anxiety. Look for others who are motivated to study hard from a desire to succeed, not from a fear of failure.

Third, reward yourself. A test is physically and mentally tiring, even without anxiety, and it can be helpful to have something to look forward to. Plan an activity following the test, regardless of the outcome, such as going to a movie or getting ice cream.

When you are taking the test, if you find yourself beginning to feel anxious, remind yourself that you know the material. Visualize successfully completing the test. Then take a few deep, relaxing breaths and return to it. Work through the questions carefully but with confidence, knowing that you are capable of succeeding.

Developing a healthy mental approach to test taking will also aid in other areas of life. Test anxiety affects more than just the actual test—it can be damaging to your mental health and even contribute to depression. It's important to beat test anxiety before it becomes a problem for more than testing.

> **Review Video: Test Anxiety and Depression**
> Visit mometrix.com/academy and enter code: 904704

171

Study Strategy

Being prepared for the test is necessary to combat anxiety, but what does being prepared look like? You may study for hours on end and still not feel prepared. What you need is a strategy for test prep. The next few pages outline our recommended steps to help you plan out and conquer the challenge of preparation.

STEP 1: SCOPE OUT THE TEST

Learn everything you can about the format (multiple choice, essay, etc.) and what will be on the test. Gather any study materials, course outlines, or sample exams that may be available. Not only will this help you to prepare, but knowing what to expect can help to alleviate test anxiety.

STEP 2: MAP OUT THE MATERIAL

Look through the textbook or study guide and make note of how many chapters or sections it has. Then divide these over the time you have. For example, if a book has 15 chapters and you have five days to study, you need to cover three chapters each day. Even better, if you have the time, leave an extra day at the end for overall review after you have gone through the material in depth.

If time is limited, you may need to prioritize the material. Look through it and make note of which sections you think you already have a good grasp on, and which need review. While you are studying, skim quickly through the familiar sections and take more time on the challenging parts. Write out your plan so you don't get lost as you go. Having a written plan also helps you feel more in control of the study, so anxiety is less likely to arise from feeling overwhelmed at the amount to cover.

STEP 3: GATHER YOUR TOOLS

Decide what study method works best for you. Do you prefer to highlight in the book as you study and then go back over the highlighted portions? Or do you type out notes of the important information? Or is it helpful to make flashcards that you can carry with you? Assemble the pens, index cards, highlighters, post-it notes, and any other materials you may need so you won't be distracted by getting up to find things while you study.

If you're having a hard time retaining the information or organizing your notes, experiment with different methods. For example, try color-coding by subject with colored pens, highlighters, or post-it notes. If you learn better by hearing, try recording yourself reading your notes so you can listen while in the car, working out, or simply sitting at your desk. Ask a friend to quiz you from your flashcards, or try teaching someone the material to solidify it in your mind.

STEP 4: CREATE YOUR ENVIRONMENT

It's important to avoid distractions while you study. This includes both the obvious distractions like visitors and the subtle distractions like an uncomfortable chair (or a too-comfortable couch that makes you want to fall asleep). Set up the best study environment possible: good lighting and a comfortable work area. If background music helps you focus, you may want to turn it on, but otherwise keep the room quiet. If you are using a computer to take notes, be sure you don't have any other windows open, especially applications like social media, games, or anything else that could distract you. Silence your phone and turn off notifications. Be sure to keep water close by so you stay hydrated while you study (but avoid unhealthy drinks and snacks).

Also, take into account the best time of day to study. Are you freshest first thing in the morning? Try to set aside some time then to work through the material. Is your mind clearer in the afternoon or evening? Schedule your study session then. Another method is to study at the same time of day that you will take the test, so that your brain gets used to working on the material at that time and will be ready to focus at test time.

STEP 5: STUDY!

Once you have done all the study preparation, it's time to settle into the actual studying. Sit down, take a few moments to settle your mind so you can focus, and begin to follow your study plan. Don't give in to distractions or let yourself procrastinate. This is your time to prepare so you'll be ready to fearlessly approach the test. Make the most of the time and stay focused.

Of course, you don't want to burn out. If you study too long you may find that you're not retaining the information very well. Take regular study breaks. For example, taking five minutes out of every hour to walk briskly, breathing deeply and swinging your arms, can help your mind stay fresh.

As you get to the end of each chapter or section, it's a good idea to do a quick review. Remind yourself of what you learned and work on any difficult parts. When you feel that you've mastered the material, move on to the next part. At the end of your study session, briefly skim through your notes again.

But while review is helpful, cramming last minute is NOT. If at all possible, work ahead so that you won't need to fit all your study into the last day. Cramming overloads your brain with more information than it can process and retain, and your tired mind may struggle to recall even previously learned information when it is overwhelmed with last-minute study. Also, the urgent nature of cramming and the stress placed on your brain contribute to anxiety. You'll be more likely to go to the test feeling unprepared and having trouble thinking clearly.

So don't cram, and don't stay up late before the test, even just to review your notes at a leisurely pace. Your brain needs rest more than it needs to go over the information again. In fact, plan to finish your studies by noon or early afternoon the day before the test. Give your brain the rest of the day to relax or focus on other things, and get a good night's sleep. Then you will be fresh for the test and better able to recall what you've studied.

STEP 6: TAKE A PRACTICE TEST

Many courses offer sample tests, either online or in the study materials. This is an excellent resource to check whether you have mastered the material, as well as to prepare for the test format and environment.

Check the test format ahead of time: the number of questions, the type (multiple choice, free response, etc.), and the time limit. Then create a plan for working through them. For example, if you have 30 minutes to take a 60-question test, your limit is 30 seconds per question. Spend less time on the questions you know well so that you can take more time on the difficult ones.

If you have time to take several practice tests, take the first one open book, with no time limit. Work through the questions at your own pace and make sure you fully understand them. Gradually work up to taking a test under test conditions: sit at a desk with all study materials put away and set a timer. Pace yourself to make sure you finish the test with time to spare and go back to check your answers if you have time.

After each test, check your answers. On the questions you missed, be sure you understand why you missed them. Did you misread the question (tests can use tricky wording)? Did you forget the information? Or was it something you hadn't learned? Go back and study any shaky areas that the practice tests reveal.

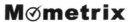

Taking these tests not only helps with your grade, but also aids in combating test anxiety. If you're already used to the test conditions, you're less likely to worry about it, and working through tests until you're scoring well gives you a confidence boost. Go through the practice tests until you feel comfortable, and then you can go into the test knowing that you're ready for it.

Test Tips

On test day, you should be confident, knowing that you've prepared well and are ready to answer the questions. But aside from preparation, there are several test day strategies you can employ to maximize your performance.

First, as stated before, get a good night's sleep the night before the test (and for several nights before that, if possible). Go into the test with a fresh, alert mind rather than staying up late to study.

Try not to change too much about your normal routine on the day of the test. It's important to eat a nutritious breakfast, but if you normally don't eat breakfast at all, consider eating just a protein bar. If you're a coffee drinker, go ahead and have your normal coffee. Just make sure you time it so that the caffeine doesn't wear off right in the middle of your test. Avoid sugary beverages, and drink enough water to stay hydrated but not so much that you need a restroom break 10 minutes into the test. If your test isn't first thing in the morning, consider going for a walk or doing a light workout before the test to get your blood flowing.

Allow yourself enough time to get ready, and leave for the test with plenty of time to spare so you won't have the anxiety of scrambling to arrive in time. Another reason to be early is to select a good seat. It's helpful to sit away from doors and windows, which can be distracting. Find a good seat, get out your supplies, and settle your mind before the test begins.

When the test begins, start by going over the instructions carefully, even if you already know what to expect. Make sure you avoid any careless mistakes by following the directions.

Then begin working through the questions, pacing yourself as you've practiced. If you're not sure on an answer, don't spend too much time on it, and don't let it shake your confidence. Either skip it and come back later, or eliminate as many wrong answers as possible and guess among the remaining ones. Don't dwell on these questions as you continue—put them out of your mind and focus on what lies ahead.

Be sure to read all of the answer choices, even if you're sure the first one is the right answer. Sometimes you'll find a better one if you keep reading. But don't second-guess yourself if you do immediately know the answer. Your gut instinct is usually right. Don't let test anxiety rob you of the information you know.

If you have time at the end of the test (and if the test format allows), go back and review your answers. Be cautious about changing any, since your first instinct tends to be correct, but make sure you didn't misread any of the questions or accidentally mark the wrong answer choice. Look over any you skipped and make an educated guess.

At the end, leave the test feeling confident. You've done your best, so don't waste time worrying about your performance or wishing you could change anything. Instead, celebrate the successful

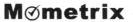

completion of this test. And finally, use this test to learn how to deal with anxiety even better next time.

Important Qualification

Not all anxiety is created equal. If your test anxiety is causing major issues in your life beyond the classroom or testing center, or if you are experiencing troubling physical symptoms related to your anxiety, it may be a sign of a serious physiological or psychological condition. If this sounds like your situation, we strongly encourage you to seek professional help.

Tell Us Your Story

We at Mometrix would like to extend our heartfelt thanks to you for letting us be a part of your journey. It is an honor to serve people from all walks of life, people like you, who are committed to building the best future they can for themselves.

We know that each person's situation is unique. But we also know that, whether you are a young student or a mother of four, you care about working to make your own life and the lives of those around you better.

That's why we want to hear your story.

We want to know why you're taking this test. We want to know about the trials you've gone through to get here. And we want to know about the successes you've experienced after taking and passing your test.

In addition to your story, which can be an inspiration both to us and to others, we value your feedback. We want to know both what you loved about our book and what you think we can improve on.

The team at Mometrix would be absolutely thrilled to hear from you! So please, send us an email at tellusyourstory@mometrix.com or visit us at mometrix.com/tellusyourstory.php and let's stay in touch.

176

Additional Bonus Material

Due to our efforts to try to keep this book to a manageable length, we've created a link that will give you access to all of your additional bonus material:

mometrix.com/bonus948/cna

Made in the USA
Las Vegas, NV
24 July 2023